THE
IDIOT'S
GUIDE

Spanish for Health Care Professionals

by Professor Richard P. Castillo
and K.D. Sullivan

ALPHA

A member of Penguin Group (USA) Inc.

Copyright © 2004 by Penguin Group (USA) Inc

Book packaging and authoring services provided by Creative Solutions Editorial, Inc.

Creative Solutions Editorial, Inc.
506 Kansas Street
San Francisco, CA 94107
800.621.2721
www.cs-edit.com

All rights reserved. No part of this book shall be reproduced, stored in a retrieval system, or transmitted by any means, electronic, mechanical, photocopying, recording, or otherwise, without written permission from the publisher. No patent liability is assumed with respect to the use of the information contained herein. Although every precaution has been taken in the preparation of this book, the publisher and authors assume no responsibility for errors or omissions. Neither is any liability assumed for damages resulting from the use of information contained herein. For information, address Alpha Books, 800 East 96th Street, Indianapolis, IN 46240.

THE POCKET IDIOT'S GUIDE TO and Design are trademarks of Penguin Group (USA) Inc.

International Standard Book Number: 978-1-59257-270-0
Library of Congress Catalog Card Number: 2004108619

13   15   14   13   12   11   10

Interpretation of the printing code: The rightmost number of the first series of numbers is the year of the book's printing; the rightmost number of the second series of numbers is the number of the book's printing. For example, a printing code of 04-1 shows that the first printing occurred in 2004.

Printed in the United States of America

Note: This publication contains the opinions and ideas of its authors. It is intended to provide helpful and informative material on the subject matter covered. It is sold with the understanding that the authors and publisher are not engaged in rendering professional services in the book. If the reader requires personal assistance or advice, a competent professional should be consulted.

The authors and publisher specifically disclaim any responsibility for any liability, loss, or risk, personal or otherwise, which is incurred as a consequence, directly or indirectly, of the use and application of any of the contents of this book.

Most Alpha books are available at special quantity discounts for bulk purchases for sales promotions, premiums, fund-raising, or educational use. Special books, or book excerpts, can also be created to fit specific needs.

For details, write: Special Markets, Alpha Books, 375 Hudson Street, New York, NY 10014.

Contents

Contents

Introduction

If you've ever been stymied by a foreign film that's not dubbed or subtitled, you can begin to appreciate how most daily encounters feel to Spanish speakers with limited English. For them, even everyday interactions can be frustrating and confusing. Imagine how those feelings can escalate to a sense of helplessness and fear when what's at stake is their health, maybe even their survival.

You are a caring professional, but if you speak only English, you are also the other half of a communication barrier. Or at least you *were*, until you picked up this book. This pocket guide will help you break down the barrier without having to spend endless hours in a night class learning how to tell someone your aunt's pen is under the table of your uncle.

The Pocket Idiot's Guide to Spanish for Health Care Professionals is a convenient, user-friendly phrase book designed to give you the words and phrases you need in your daily work, packaged in useful sentences and phonetically transcribed to make even your first stab at communication successful. To make it even easier, lead-in phrases and a choice of completions let you form just the sentence you need.

We hope you'll read the whole book, of course; but if your time is at a premium, go right to the phrases you need. As you scan the page for what you have in mind, don't overlook the helpful reminders and cultural insights called "¡Ojo!" (the Spanish word for eye, which can also mean heads up, watch out, pay attention) and "Through Their Eyes."

Although not intended to be a comprehensive language guide, the first two chapters of this book provide a brief user's guide, language primer, and collection of words and phrases common to many different situations. Subsequent chapters deal with specific areas, such as welcoming, examining, diagnosing, treating, surgery, emergencies, and others, where language structures are familiar, but the vocabulary is more restricted.

With *The Pocket Idiot's Guide to Spanish for Health Care Professionals* you can break the communication barrier and establish a closer relationship with your Spanish-speaking patients. You can offer them reassurance, information, and ultimately better-quality care. You'll also make more efficient use of your own time. So ...

Shall we go on?   ¿Continuamos?   kohn tee
NWAH mohs

Acknowledgments

This guide, from concept to reality, has been a collaborative effort. So we're grateful to each other; without the vital contribution of each member of the team, this book would have remained just a good idea. The authors also wish to express sincere gratitude to our ever-patient companions—both two- and four-legged—for their unwavering support, with special thanks to Jere and Robert.

Dedication

Dedicated to those health care professionals who
have purchased this book in an attempt to communicate effectively and respectfully with their
Spanish-speaking patients.

Trademarks

All terms mentioned in this book that are known to
be or are suspected of being trademarks or service
marks have been appropriately capitalized. Alpha
Books and Penguin Group (USA) Inc. cannot attest
to the accuracy of this information. Use of a term
in this book should not be regarded as affecting the
validity of any trademark or service mark.

Spanish from the Ground Up

The words and phrases in this guide will open new worlds of communication between you and your Spanish-speaking patients. But before you get to them, spend a few minutes with this chapter, learning the building blocks of the language, so you'll understand how those phrases are formed and be more confident forming and saying your own. Compared to English, Spanish can be refreshingly uncomplicated; after you know the basics, you'll be feeling bilingual in no time.

Same Alphabet, New Sounds

In English, the connection between spelling and pronunciation can be a little, well, *distant*. To say nothing of fickle. In Spanish, spelling is a much more trustworthy guide to pronunciation. There's far more consistency in Spanish; if you know the Spanish sounds for the letters, and which syllable to stress, you'll know how to pronounce any written word.

Spanish is spoken by 400 million people in 23 countries worldwide, so as you'd expect, pronunciation isn't *entirely* consistent. But don't worry. The pronunciations shown in this guide are in what's called Universal Standard Spanish, which has no regional quirks and is understood by all Spanish speakers. The stressed syllables are shown in capital letters (more about that in a bit).

Vowels Are Vital

More than anything else, Spanish vowels are what give the language its distinctive sound. Learning to pronounce them correctly is the best and easiest thing you can do to help your patients understand you. Each has one sound only, even when two vowels appear together.

Vowel	Sound	Example
a	ah (as in yacht)	asma /AHS mah/ asthma
e	eh (as in place)	este /EHS teh/ this
i	ee (as in meet)	sí /see/ yes
o	oh (as in go)	ojo /OH hoh/ eye
u	oo (as in glue)	sutura /soo TOO rah/ suture
u (after *Q*)	silent	quiste /KEES teh/ cyst

Diphthongs—When Vowels Meet

Each vowel in Spanish forms its own syllable, and when a word contains back-to-back vowels, each one keeps its own sound. For instance:

deseo
deh SEH oh
I would like

The vowels *I* and *U*, however, combine with other vowels to create a single syllable voiced with a connecting sound. For the *I* combinations, that sound is a *Y*; for the *U*, it is a *W*.

Diphthong	Sound	Example
ai	ay (as in eye)	aire /AY reh/ air
ia	yah (as in yacht)	anemia /ah NEH myah/ anemia
au	ow (as in trout)	trauma /TROW mah/ trauma
ua	wah (as in walk)	cuando /KWAHN doh/ when
ie	yeh (as in yes)	hielo /HYEH loh/ ice
ei	ey (as in feign)	veinte /BEYN teh/ twenty
eu	ehw (as in feud but no Y sound)	neurosis /nehw ROH sees/ neurosis
ue	weh (as in wait)	hueso /WEH soh/ bone
oi	oy (as in boy)	voy /boy/ I'm going
io	yoh (as in yo-yo)	erupción /eh roop SYOHN/ rash
ui	wee (as in we)	cuidado /kwee THAH thoh/ care
iu	yoo (as in you)	diurético /dyoo REH tee koh/ diuretic

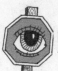

¡Ojo!

The *u* in *que* and *qui* is always silent; and the *u* in *gue* and *gui* is silent unless it has two dots over it:

ataque /ah TAH keh/ attack
quiste /KEES teh/ cyst
distingue /dees TEENG geh/ distinguish
guía /GEE ah/ guide (book)
vergüenza /behr GWEHN sah/ shame

Constant Consonants

The remainder of the sounds in Spanish come from the consonants. With a few exceptions and additions, they are pronounced the same in Spanish as in English. The consonants are easy to learn, and best of all, they're consistent.

Consonant	Sound	Example
b	b (as in box)	boca /BOH kah/ mouth
	v (as in view, softened)	labio /LAH vyoh/ lip

(*B* has two sounds, determined by the letters that surround it. In transcriptions, you'll see it sometimes one way and sometimes the other.)

c (before *E* or *I*)	s (as in Sam)	cintura /seen TOO rah/ waist
c (elsewhere)	k (as in like)	cabeza /kah VEH sah/ head
ch	ch (as in check)	choque /CHOH keh/ shock

Consonant	Sound	Example
d	d (as in dog, softened)	dedo /DEH thoh/ finger
	th (as in bathe)	dedo /DEH thoh/ finger

(*D* has two sounds, determined by the letters that surround it. In transcriptions, you'll see it sometimes one way and sometimes the other.)

f	f (as in first, not of)	feto /FEH toh/ fetus
g (before *E* or *I*)	h (gargled sound, as in Lo*ch* Ness, *Ch*anukah, and the German na*ch*t)	gente /HEHN teh/ people
g (elsewhere)	g (as in good, softened)	agua /AH gwah/ water
h	(silent)	hora /OH rah/ hour
j	h (same as gargled *G*)	jeringa /heh REEN gah/ syringe
k	k (as in like)	kilo /KEE loh/ kilo
l	l (as in let)	leche /LEH cheh/ milk
ll	y (as in kayak)	callo /KAH yoh/ callus
m	m (as in more)	más /MAHS/ more
n	n (as in nothing)	nada /NAH thah/ nothing
ñ	ny (as in bunion)	baño /BAHN yoh/ bath(room)
p	p (as in pie, softened)	para /PAH rah/ for

continues

continued

Consonant	Sound	Example
q	k (as in like)	queso /KEH soh/ cheese
r (at beg. of a word)	rr (rolled r)	raro /RRAH roh/ rare
r (elsewhere)	r (with a slight D sound added, as in bird)	cara /KAH rah/ face
rr	rr (rolled r)	carro /KAH rroh/ car
s	s (as in so)	sed /SEHTH/ thirst(y)
t	t (as in true, softened)	tos /TOHS/ cough
v	b (as in baby, softened)	visita /bee SEE tah/ visit
w	w (as in water; only in words borrowed from other languages)	Wasserman /WAH sehr mahn
x (followed by a vowel)	ks (as in taxi)	taxi /TAHK see/ taxi
x (elsewhere)	s (as in Sam)	extra /EHS trah/ extra
y (the word)	ee (as in tea)	café y té /kah FEH ee TEH/ coffee and tea
y (all other)	y (as in yes)	yerba /YEHR vah/ grass or herb
z	s (as in Sam)	bazo /BAH soh/ spleen

¡Ojo!

The mark over the *N* in a word like *baño* is small but very important. *Uña* = fingernail, but *una* = one; *año* = year, but *ano* = anus; *cono* = cone, but *coño* = cunt.

Spelling It Out

The *sounds* of the letters are one thing; their *names* are another. In talking with patients, you may need to spell a word out, letter for letter, so you'll need to know how to pronounce the names of the letters in Spanish.

When You Need to Spell It Out

Letter	Pronunciation
a	ah
b	beh GRAHN deh (to distinguish from *V*)
c	seh
ch*	cheh
d	deh
e	eh
f	EH feh
g	heh
h	AH cheh
i	ee

continues

When You Need to Spell It Out   (continued)

Letter	Pronunciation
j	HO tah
k	kah
l	EH leh
ll*	EH yeh *or* dohs EH lehs
m	EH meh
n	EH neh
ñ	EH nyeh
o	oh
p	peh
q	koo
r	EH reh
rr	EH rreh *or* dohs EH rrehs
s	EH seh
t	teh
u	oo
v	beh CHEE kah (to distinguish from *B*)
w	DOH bleh beh
x	EH kees
y	ee gree EH gah
z	SEH tah

These letters, as units, are no longer part of the official Spanish alphabet, but Spanish speakers still use their names when spelling out a word.

Stress Is a Good Thing

After you know the sounds, the only thing between you and good Spanish pronunciation is knowing which syllables to stress as you speak them. You can let the capital letters shown in this book guide you, or you can rely on three hard-and-fast rules:

Rule 1. If the word has a written accent mark (´), stress the syllable with the mark:

dirección	dee rehk SYOHN	address, direction
úlcera	OOL seh rah	ulcer
práctico	PRAHK tee koh	practical
practicó	prahk tee KOH	he practiced

Rule 2. If the word carries no accent mark and ends with a vowel (*A, E, I, O, U*), or an *N* or *S*, stress the next-to-last syllable:

resfriado	rrehs FRYAH thoh	head cold
rodillas	rroh THEE yahs	knees
vienen	BYEH nehn	they come
practico	prahk TEE koh	I practice

Rule 3. If the word carries no accent mark and ends with any consonant *other* than *N* or *S*, stress the last syllable:

comer	koh MEHR	to eat
vegetal	beh heh TAHL	vegetable

| habilidad | ah vee lee THAHTH | ability |
| feliz | feh LEES | happy |

¡Ojo!

English speakers often think Spanish speakers talk quickly. But it's not speed you hear, it's linking. When one word ends with a vowel and the next begins with one, Spanish speakers join the two to pronounce what sounds like a single word. In this guide, you'll see underscores to indicate linking:

¿Cómo está usted hoy?
KOH moh_ehs TAH_oos TEHTH oy
How are you today?

An Agreeable Language

English nouns have only two forms, singular and plural: man/men, tree/trees, woman/women, test/tests. And face it, except biologically speaking, they are sexless. Words referring to either form have only one form: the old … man (men), tree(s), woman (women), test(s).

In Spanish, however, singular and plural nouns—even inanimate ones!—have sex, and the words that hang around with them do, too.

For Every Noun, a Gender

When you learn the Spanish word for a person, place, or thing, you must learn its gender at the same time. The article that precedes it will clue you in.

	The (Singular)	The (Plural)	A, An, One	Some
Masculine	el	los	un	unos
Feminine	la	las	una	unas

You can also often tell the gender of a noun by its ending. Nouns that end in *O* are usually masculine; nouns that end in *A* are usually feminine.

el cuello	ehl KWEH oh	the neck
los ojos	lohs OH hohs	the eyes
un labio	oon LAH vyoh	a lip
unos órganos	OO nohs OHR gah nohs	some organs
la cabeza	lah kah VEH sah	the head
las orejas	lahs oh REH hahs	the ears
una cita	OO nah SEE tah	an appointment
unas alergias	OO nahs ah LEHR hyahs	some allergies

There are a few exceptions to this rule, and there are also nouns that don't end in either *O* or *A*. These you'll just need to memorize, but it's not a big task.

¡Ojo!

Some Spanish nouns can change gender depending on the sex of the person referred to:

el doctor
ehl dohk TOHR
the (male) doctor

la doctora
lah dohk TOHR ah
the (female) doctor

Others keep their gender no matter whom they refer to:

el bebé
ehl beh VEH
baby, the baby

la persona
lah pehr SOHN ah
person, the person

That Goes for Adjectives, Too

In Spanish, words that describe people, places, and things also change based on gender and number. Here's a masculine example:

el diente blanco
ehl DYEHN teh BLAHN koh
the white tooth

un diente blanco
oon DYEHN teh BLAHN koh
a white tooth

los dientes blancos
lohs DYEHN tehs BLAHN kohs
the white teeth

unos dientes blancos
OO nohs DYEHN tehs BLAHN kohs
some white teeth

And a feminine example:

la venda blanca
lah BEHN dah BLAHN kah
the white bandage

una venda blanca
OO nah BEHN dah BLAHN kah
a white bandage

las vendas blancas
lahs BEHN dahs BLAHN kas
the white bandages

unas vendas blancas
OO nahs BEHN dahs BLAHN kas
some white bandages

This gender bending and number crunching is really pretty simple. The following ending guidelines will keep most nouns and adjectives in perfect agreement. Create the different forms this way.

All's Well That Ends Well

For Words Ending in O		
	Singular	*Plural*
Masculine	no change	-s
Feminine	-a	-as

All's Well That Ends Well   (continued)

For Words Ending in Another Vowel

	Singular	Plural
Masculine	no change	-s
Feminine	no change	-s

For Words Ending in a Consonant

	Singular	Plural
Masculine	no change	-es
Feminine	no change	no change

See how *roto* (broken), *permanente* (permanent), and *topical* (topical) change in these phrases:

> unas costillas rotas
> OO nahs kohs TEE yahs RROH tahs
> some broken ribs
>
> unas marcas permanentes
> OO nahs MAHR kahs pehr mah NEHN tehs
> some permanent marks
>
> unos ungüentos topicales
> OO nohs oon GWEHN tohs toh pee KAH lehs
> some topical ointments

The Order of Things

There's one other thing about Spanish descriptors, and you've probably already noticed it. In English, adjectives usually precede the word they describe. In Spanish, they usually come after it:

> una puerta grande
> OO nah PWEHR tah GRAHN deh
> a big door

> el té frío
> ehl teh FREE oh
> cold tea

Location, Location, Location

Frequently, you'll want to describe a thing by indicating its location. Like other adjectives, the pointing words—this, these, that, and those—must agree with the noun.

The Pointing Words

	This	These
Masculine	este /EHS teh	estos /EHS tohs
Feminine	esta /EHS tah	estas /EHS tahs
	that (nearby)	**those (nearby)**
Masculine	ese /EHS eh	esos /EHS ohs
Feminine	esa /EHS ah	esas /EHS ahs
	that (distant)	**those (distant)**
Masculine	aquel /ah KEHL	aquellos /ah KEH yohs
Feminine	aquella /ah KEHL ah	aquellas /ah KEH yahs

¡Ojo!

Unlike other adjectives, the locator words come *before* the word they describe, just as you'd place them in English:

este cuarto
EHS teh KWAHR toh
this room

esos libros
EH sohs LEE vrohs
those books

aquel hospital
ah KEHL ohs pee TAHL
that hospital

What's Yours and What's Mine

Another way to indicate which one is to say whose it is: your name, my car, his coat, and so on. By now it should come as no surprise that in Spanish, these possessives don't exist in a vacuum. They must agree with the thing possessed, *not*—careful here—*the possessor*. However, with one exception (our), gender is not a factor; the forms change only between singular and plural.

So it's ...

mi esposo	mee ehs POH soh	my husband
mi esposa	mee ehs POH sah	my wife

And it's ...

su hija	soo EE hah	your daughter

but …

nuestras	NWEHS trahs	our
hijas	EE hahs	daughters

Possessives: Whose Is It?

Possessive	Singular	Plural
my	mi /mee	mis /mees
your (familiar)	tu /too	tus /toos
his, her, your (polite), its, their	su /soo	sus /soos
our	nuestro /noo EHS troh	nuestros / noo EHS trohs
	nuestra /noo EHS trah	nuestras /noo EHS trahs

Who's Doing It?

Before you set your Spanish in motion with verbs, you must know who or what is performing the action. In Spanish, as in English, that's the subject of a sentence—a noun or a pronoun. Here are the Spanish subject pronouns.

Subject Pronoun	Singular	Plural
I, we	yo /yoh	nosotros /noh SOH trohs
we (f.)	nosotras / noh SOH trahs	

continues

continued

Subject Pronoun	Singular	Plural
you (familiar)	tú /too	—
you (polite)	usted /oo STETH	ustedes /oos TEH thehs
he, they (m)	él /ehl	ellos /EH yohs
she, they (f)	ella /EH yah	ellas /EH yahs

In Spanish, the pronoun "you" has shades of meaning not found in English. Use *tú* when speaking to a child or a close friend or relative; use *usted* or *ustedes* (often shortened to *Ud.* or *Uds.*) when speaking to anyone else. And there's still another form of "you"—*vosostros*—that's used primarily in Spain. In this guide, we'll stick to *usted*.

Note that for groups of women, there are special forms of "we" and "they," but the same plural "you" is used for both men and women.

¡Ojo!

Because every Spanish noun has a gender, there is no subject word for "it."

When English uses this neuter pronoun as the subject of a sentence, Spanish uses the verb alone, in the "he/she" form, with no pronoun at all:

It works like this.
Funciona así.
foon SYOH nah_ah SEE

The Invisible Pronoun

In English, the pronoun tells you "who" does the action. In Spanish, because the form of the verb already indicates the subject, pronouns are very often dropped. So ...

> Usted necesita volver.
> oos TEHTH neh seh SEE tah BOHL behr
> You need to come back.

can become ...

> Necesita volver.
> neh seh SEE tah BOHL behr

And ...

> ¿Tiene usted alguna pregunta?
> TYEH neh_oos TEHTH ahl GOO nah preh GOON tah
> Do you have any questions?

can become ...

> ¿Tiene alguna pregunta?
> TYEH neh_ahl GOO nah preh GOON tah

¡Ojo!

When Spanish subject pronouns are used, they generally precede the verb in statements and follow it in questions.

Who's Receiving It?

Spanish pronouns change form when they're receiving the action rather than performing it; that is, when they're objects rather than subjects.

Here are the pronouns to use on the receiving end.

Object Pronoun	Singular	Plural
me, us	me /meh	nos /nohs
you (familiar)	te /teh	—
you (polite)	lo /loh	los /lohs
	la /lah	las /lahs
him, them	lo /loh	los /lohs
her, them	la /lah	las /lahs

For example:

> Yo lo comprendo pero ¿me comprende usted?
> yoh loh kohm PREHN doh PEH roh meh
> kohm PREHN deh_oos TEHTH
> I understand you, but do you understand me?

Me, Myself, and I

Sometimes the subject is also the receiver of the action. As in, "I hurt myself." In English, it takes a special type of pronoun to make that point: the reflexive. Myself, yourself, himself, themselves … all these "self" pronouns toss the action back to the subject, where it began.

Spanish also has a set of reflexive pronouns, as follows.

Subject	Reflexive	Subject	Reflexive
yo	me	nosotros (-as)	nos
tú	te	—	—
él	se	ellos	se
ella	se	ellas	se
usted	se	ustedes	se

Most often, the reflexive is used in Spanish to convey the English sense of "get" or "become":

> Ella *se* levanta.
> EH yah seh leh VAHN tah
> She gets up. (stands up)
>
> enfermar*se*
> ehn fehr MAHR seh
> to get sick
>
> *Me* enfermo si como mariscos.
> meh ehn FEHR moh see KOH moh mah REES kohs
> I get sick if I eat seafood.
>
> No quiero enfermar*me*.
> noh KYEH roh_ehn fehr MAHR meh
> I don't want to get sick.

In all these examples, note the placement of the reflexive pronoun. Generally, object pronouns precede a conjugated verb and follow a command or an unconjugated verb.

Add Action with Verbs

In Spanish, as in English, all verbs start as infinitives, the "to" form of the verb. *Hablar* (to speak), *comer* (to eat), *escribir* (to write). From there, the endings change to fit the subject and time frame. *Yo hablo* (I speak), *usted habla* (you speak), *ellas hablan* (they speak). *How* they change depends on the type of verb.

Rely on the Regulars

In Spanish, most verbs are *regular*, meaning the changes to their endings are consistent and predictable. After you know the scheme, you can apply it to any verb of the same type.

There are just three large groups of regular Spanish verbs, infinitives ending in *–AR*, *–ER*, and *–IR*. Here are some examples.

Some Common Regular Verbs

-AR Verbs		
buscar	boos KAHR	to look for
escuchar	ehs koo CHAHR	to listen to
llegar	yeh GAHR	to arrive
regresar	reh greh SAHR	to return
tomar	toh MAHR	to take

-ER Verbs		
beber	beh VEHR	to drink
depender	deh pehn DEHR	to depend
leer	leh EHR	to read
proceder	proh seh THEHR	to proceed
responder	reh spohn DEHR	to respond

-IR Verbs		
abrir	ah VREEHR	to open
decidir	deh see THEER	to decide
salir	sah LEER	to go out
prevenir	preh beh NEER	to prevent
vivir	bee VEER	to live

Conjugate with Confidence

Each of the regular verb types in Spanish is conjugated according to strict patterns. If you know a verb's family connections, you can tailor it to fit any context, based on the rules for that type of verb. The patterns indicate …

- **The person.** Who's performing the action: I, you, he, she, they, and so on.
- **The tense.** When the action takes place: past, present, future, and versions thereof.

The number of tenses in Spanish would turn this *Pocket Idiot's Guide* into a weighty grammar book; the few you see here are the ones you'll use most often.

The Present

You work, You do work, You are working
Usted trabaja
oos TEHTH trah BAH hah

Conjugation: Who's Doing It Now?

Subject	-AR Verbs	-ER Verbs	-IR Verbs
	(*tomar*)	(*beber*)	(*vivir*)
yo	tomo	bebo	vivo
tú	tomas	bebes	vives
él, ella, Ud.	toma	bebe	vive
nosotros	tomamos	bebemos	vivimos
ellos, ellas, Uds.	toman	beben	viven

The Completed Past

You worked, You did work
Usted trabajó
oos TEHTH trah vah HOH

Conjugation: Who Already Did It?

Subject	-AR Verbs	-ER Verbs	-IR Verbs
	(*tomar*)	(*beber*)	(*vivir*)
yo	tomé	bebí	viví
tú	tomaste	bebiste	viviste
lla, Ud.	tomó	bebió	vivió
ros	tomamos	bebimos	vivimos
llas, Uds.	tomaron	bebieron	vivieron

The Descriptive Past

You were working, You used to work
Usted trabajaba
oos TEHTH trah vah HAH vah

Conjugation: Who Was Doing It or Used to Do It?

Subject	-AR Verbs	-ER Verbs	-IR Verbs
	(*tomar*)	(*beber*)	(*vivir*)
yo	tomaba	bebía	vivía
tú	tomabas	bebías	vivías
él, ella, Ud.	tomaba	bebía	vivía
nosotros	tomábamos	bebíamos	vivíamos
ellos, ellas, Uds.	tomaban	bebían	vivían

The Conditional

You would work
Usted trabajaría
oos TEHTH trah vah hahr EE ah

¡Ojo!

For this tense, there is just one set of endings for all three verb families, and they attach to the entire infinitive.

Conjugation: Who Would Do It?

Subject	-AR Verbs	-ER Verbs	-IR Verbs
	(*tomar*)	(*beber*)	(*vivir*)
yo	tomaría	bebería	viviría
tú	tomarías	beberías	vivirías
él, ella, Ud.	tomaría	bebería	viviría
nosotros	tomaríamos	beberíamos	viviríamos
ellos, ellas, Uds.	tomarían	beberían	vivirían

In the next chapter, you'll see how these elements combine to form phrases you can start using right away.

Chapter 2

Communication Basics

This chapter contains the words and phrases you'll use most often with your Spanish-speaking patients. First, you'll learn greetings and courtesies to put patients at ease, and how to interact with them in ways that gain trust and cooperation. Then you'll learn everyday vocabulary useful in any medical setting.

Greetings

The way you greet a patient can set the tone for the entire visit. Make a good first impression by using the language he or she knows best. Even if you falter or slip back into English, Spanish speakers will appreciate your effort.

Here are the most basic greetings:

Hello./Hi.	Hola.	OH lah
Good morning.	Buenos días.	BWEH nohs THEE ahs
Good afternoon.	Buenas tardes.	BWEH nahs TAHR thehs
Good evening.	Buenas tardes.	BWEH nahs TAR thehs

¡Ojo!

Hola is as casual and informal as "Hi," so use the other greetings until the patient uses *Hola* with you first.

Spanish speakers use *días* until noon, then *tardes* for the remainder of the day and evening. *Buenas noches,* like its English counterpart "Good night," is a farewell, not a greeting.

Through Their Eyes

It's common to combine *Hola* with any of the other greetings while extending the hand for a handshake. This does not sound as redundant in Spanish as "Hello, good morning" does in English.

Follow a greeting with a friendly question that shows your concern and starts the flow of information:

How are you, ma'am?
¿Cómo está usted, señora?
KOH mo_ehs TAH_oos TEHTH seh
NYOH rah

sir?	señor?	seh NYOHR
young man?	joven?	HOH vehn
miss?	señorita?	seh nyoh REE tah
young lady?	señorita?	seh nyoh REE tah
my little man?	mi hijo?	mee_EE hoh
my little lady?	mi hija?	mee_EE hah

These simple forms of address are very powerful tools. Using them shows respect, both to the patient and family members, and will win you respect in return.

Through Their Eyes

Joven is an especially important word to Spanish speakers; it acknowledges a boy's transition to manhood. Addressing a teenager this way will work wonders! The same is true, to a lesser degree, for *señorita*. And if you know an adult's family name, add it to show even more respect:

¡Buenos días! ¿Cómo está usted, señora Cornejo?
BWEH nos THEE ahs, KOH moh_ ehs TAH_oos TEHTH, seh NYOH rah kohr NEH hoh

When you're more familiar with your patients, you can greet them less formally:

Hi, Rogelio! How are things?
¡Hola Rogelio! ¿Qué tal?
OH lah rroh HEH lyoh, keh tahl

How's it going?
¿Cómo le va?
KOH moh leh vah

Show your respect for familiar seniors by adding *don* to a man's first name and *doña* to a woman's:

> Hi, Carlos. How are things?
> Hola, don Carlos. ¿Qué tal?
> OH lah thohn KAHR lohs, keh tahl

> Hi, Maria. What's been up with you?
> Hola, doña María. ¿Qué me cuenta?
> OH lah DOH nyah mah REE ah keh meh
> KWEHN tah

More Courtesies

To round out your interactions with Spanish-speaking patients, here are a few more civilities:

Please	Por favor	pohr fah VOHR
Thank you	Gracias	GRAH syahs
You're welcome	De nada	deh NAH thah
Excuse me (to take leave or pass by people)	Permiso	pehr MEE soh
I'm sorry (to request forgiveness at the time for hurting, interrupting, offending, etc.)	Perdón	pehr THOHN
I'm sorry (to make amends afterwards for having hurt, interrupted, offended, etc.)	Lo siento	loh SYEHN toh
Good-bye	Adiós	ah THYOHS

Asking Questions

To help patients, you must gather information. Here are some simple questions you'll use often:

How many?	¿Cuántos(as)?	KWAHN tohs(tahs)
How much?	¿Cuánto(a)?	KWAHN toh(tah)
How? (asks for condition or manner)	¿Cómo?	KOH moh
What? (identification or label)	¿Qué?	keh
What for? (asks the purpose or goal)	¿Para qué?	PAH rah keh
What time? (a more specific "When?")	¿A qué hora?	ah keh_OH rah
When? (a general "When?")	¿Cuándo?	KWAHN doh
Which? (thing)	¿Qué?	keh
Which? (one[s])	¿Cuál(es)?	kwahl (KWAH lehs)
Who?	¿Quién(es)?	kyehn (KYEH nehs)
Why? (asks the reason or cause)	¿Por qué?	pohr keh

To form other questions, follow these guidelines:

To ask a question that can be answered by "yes" or "no," put the subject after the verb and be sure to raise your pitch at the end.

Can you ... ?	¿Puede usted ... ?	PWEH theh_ oos TEHTH ...

To verify if something is the case, make a normally intoned statement, and then add a positive *¿verdad?* /behr THAHTH/ or a negative *¿no?* tag with the rising pitch of a question.

> You understand me, don't you?
> Usted me comprende, ¿verdad?
> oos TEHTH meh kohm PREHN deh,
> vehr THAHTH

Manners Matter

You know that *how* you ask a question is often as important as *what* you ask. This is especially true when caring for Spanish-speaking patients. When you seek information deferentially, rather than demand it, you'll gain far better trust and cooperation. The verbs *poder* (can, be able) and *querer* (to want) will help you form gentler questions.

For example, instead of asking a personal question such as "How old are you?" directly ...

> ¿Cuántos años tiene usted?
> KWAHN tohs AH nyohs TYEH neh_oos
> TEHTH

soften it with the polite form:

> Can you/Do you want to tell me how old you are?
> ¿Puede/Quiere decirme su edad?
> PWEH theh/KYEH reh theh SEER meh soo_eh
> THAHTH

A simpler approach is to form the question without using *poder* or *querer* at all:

> (Literally) Are you saying your age for me?
> ¿Me dice su edad?
> meh DEE seh soo_eh THAHTH

¡Ojo!

For English speakers, it's tempting to simply use the Spanish for "please," *por favor,* as an all-purpose way to soften requests. An occasional *por favor* is fine, but using too many sounds artificial. Instead, imitate native speakers by using *quisiera* and *pudiera.*

Assuring Candor

Some patients who have trouble understanding your Spanish may—out of politeness and respect for you—try to avoid telling you they don't understand, answering your questions with a tentative, noncommittal *sí,* or whatever they believe you want to hear. The gentlest way to achieve candid communication is to say ...

> It's important that we understand each other.
> Es importante que nos comprendamos.
> ehs eem pohr TAHN teh keh nohs kohm prehn DAH mohs

Don't hesitate to ask if you have a question.
No deje de hacerme pregunta si tiene alguna duda.
noh THEH heh theh_ah SEHR meh preh
GOON tah see TYEH neh_ahl GOO nah
THOO thah

And lay your own cards out on the table; don't be
afraid to solicit their help:

I'm sorry, I don't understand …
Disculpe, no comprendo …
dees KOOL peh noh kohm PREHN doh

Could you … ?
¿Puede …
PWEH theh …

repeat that?
repetirlo?
reh peh TEER loh

say that more slowly?
decirlo más despacio?
theh SEER loh mahs dehs PAH syoh

say it another way?
decirlo de otra manera
theh SEER loh theh_OH trah mah NEH rah

Giving Instructions

The most direct (but also the harshest) way to give
instructions is the command:

You have to take this with food.
Tiene que tomar esto con comida.
TYEH neh keh toh MAHR EHS toh kohn koh
MEE thah

In some situations, such as emergencies, it's necessary to use an even more terse form:

> Hold on to the rail.
> ¡Agarre usted la barra!
> ah GAH rreh_oo STETH lah BAH rrah

To form a direct command, mentally create the present tense *yo* form of the verb, then replace the final
O with an *E* if the infinitve was *–AR*, or with an *A*
if the infinitive was *–ER* or *–IR*. If this seems a bit
messy, start memorizing these common commands.

True Commands: When You Need to Get It Done

Verb	Command (*Usted*)	
bend	flexione	flehk SYOH neh
calm down	cálmese	KAHL meh seh
close	cierre	SYEH rreh
come	venga	BEHN gah
cough	tosa	TOH sah
do	haga	AH gah
exhale	espire	ehs SPEE reh
get down	bájese	BAH heh seh
get on	súbase	SOO vah seh
give	dé	deh
go	vaya	BAH yah
hold (it)	aguante	ah GWAHN teh
inhale	aspire	ah SPEE reh
lie down	échese	EH cheh seh
listen	escuche	ehs KOO cheh

continues

True Commands: When You Need to Get It Done (continued)

Verb	Command (*Usted*)	
look	mire	MEE reh
lower	baje	BAH heh
make	haga	AH gah
open	abra	AH vrah
put on	póngase	POHN gah seh
raise	levante	leh VAHN teh
relax	relájese	rreh LAH heh seh
say	diga	DEE gah
show	muestre	MWEHS treh
sit	siéntese	SYEHN teh seh
stand	párese	PAH reh seh
take off	quítese	KEE teh seh
take	tome	TOH meh
tell	diga	DEE gah
turn	vuelva	BWEHL bah

For the *Ustedes* command, just add a final *N* to the *Usted* version.

Normally, however, a litany of direct commands can be offensive, and especially so to Spanish speakers. So unless the situation is urgent, try to use one of the gentler request forms shown in the previous section.

Vocabulary for All

The lists in this section contain words and phrases commonly used in a variety of medical settings. More specialized vocabulary appears in the chapters that follow.

¡Ojo!
You'll soon find there are some words and phrases you need more often than others. For quick reference, create your own custom crib sheet and keep it handy.

Family

Family is very important in the Hispanic world. Here are the words that describe family relationships. The masculine plural forms automatically include the feminine, so *hijos* means "sons" or "sons and daughters."

Men	Hombres	OHM brehs
cousin	primo	PREE moh
dad	papá	pah PAH
father	padre	PAH threh
father-in-law	suegro	SWE groh
grandfather	abuelo	a VWEH loh
husband	esposo	ehs POH soh
husband	marido	mah REE thoh
nephew	sobrino	soh VREE noh

continues

continued

Men	Hombres	OHM brehs
fiancé	novio	NOH vyoh
partner	compañero	kohm pah NYEH roh
son	hijo	EE hoh
son-in-law	yerno	YEHR noh
uncle	tío	TEE oh

Women	Mujeres	moo HEH rehs
aunt	tía	TEE ah
cousin	prima	PREE mah
daughter	hija	EE hah
daughter-in-law	nuera	NWEH rah
grandmother	abuela	a VWEH lah
fiancée	novia	NOH vyah
mom	mamá	mah MAH
mother	madre	MAH THREH
mother-in-law	suegra	SWEH grah
niece	sobrina	soh VREE nah
partner	compañera	kohm pah NYEH rah
wife	esposa	ehs POH sah
wife	mujer	moo HEHR

Staff Members

assistant	ayudante	ah yoo DAHN teh
dietician	dietista	dyeh TEES tah
doctor	doctor	dohk TOHR
nurse	enfermera	ehn fehr MEH rah

orderly	practicante	prahk tee KAHN teh
pharmacist	farmacéutico	fahr mah SEHW tee koh
technician	técnico	TEHK nee koh
therapist	terapeuta	teh rah PEHW tah

Sensations

In English, these phrases are used with the verb "to be." In Spanish, they're expressed with forms of the irregular verb *tener* (to have):

yo	tengo	TEHN goh
tú	tienes	TYEH nehs
él, ella, Ud.	tiene	TYEH neh
nosotros	tenemos	teh NEH mohs
ellos, ellas, Uds.	tienen	TYEH nehn
to be …	tener …	teh NEHR
(very) hot	(mucho) calor	kah LOHR
(very) cold	(mucho) frío	FREE oh
(very) sleepy	(mucho) sueño	SWEH nyoh
(very) hungry	(mucha) hambre	AHM breh
(very) scared	(mucho) miedo	MYEH thoh
(not very) thirsty	(poca) sed	sehth
(very) in a hurry	(mucha) prisa	PREE sah
(so) embarrassed	(tanta) vergüenza	vehr GWEHN sah

To express inclination and obligation, also use *tener*:

> to feel like [-ing]
> ganas de [infinitive]
> GAH nahs theh
>
> to have to [infinitive]
> que [infinitive]
> keh
>
> Do you feel like sleeping now?
> ¿Tiene ganas de dormir ahora?
> TYEH neh GAH nahs theh thohr MEER ah_OH rah
>
> You have to keep this dry.
> Tiene que mantenerlo seco.
> TYEH neh keh mahn teh NEHR loh SEH koh

Emotional States

These are considered a state, *estado*, of affairs, so they are expressed with the irregular verb *estar*:

yo	estoy	ehs TOY
tú	estás	ehs TAHS
él, ella, Ud.	está	ehs TAH
nosotros	estamos	ehs TAH mohs
ellos, ellas, Uds.	están	ehs TAHN

Yo estoy …

angry	enojado	eh noh HAH thoh
bored	aburrido	ah voo RREE thoh
calm	calmado	kahl MAH thoh
confused	confundido	kohn foon DEE thoh
excited	emocionado	eh moh syoh NAH thoh

happy	feliz	feh LEES
mad	enojado	eh noh HAH thoh
relaxed	relajado	rreh lah HAH thoh
sad	triste	trees teh
startled	espantado	ehs pahn TAH thoh
surprised	sorprendido	sohr prehn DEE thoh
worried	preocupado	preh oh koo PAH thoh

Days of the Week

Monday	el lunes	ehl LOO nehs
Tuesday	el martes	ehl MAHR tehs
Wednesday	el miércoles	ehl MYEHR koh lehs
Thursday	el jueves	ehl HWEH vehs
Friday	el viernes	ehl VYEHR nehs
Saturday	el sábado	ehl SAH vah thoh
Sunday	el domingo	ehl thoh MEEN goh

The articles *el* (singular) and *los* (plural) are always used with the days of the week, rather than such words as *this, next, last, on, by,* or *every.* To form the plural, add an *S* to *sábado* and *domingo;* the other days do not change:

by Friday	el viernes
last Thursday	el jueves
on Tuesdays	los martes
every Sunday	los domingos

In addition to the names of the days, there are other ways to refer to them:

the day before yesterday	anteayer	ahn teh ah YEHR
yesterday	ayer	ah YEHR
today	hoy	oy
tomorrow	mañana	mah NYAH nah
the day after tomorrow	pasado mañana	pah SAH thoh mah NYAH nah
the weekend	el fin de semana	ehl feen deh seh MAH nah
weekends	los fines de semana	lohs FEE nehs theh seh MAH nah

Months and Seasons

January	enero	eh NEH roh
February	febrero	feh VREH roh
March	marzo	MAHR soh
April	abril	ah VREEL
May	mayo	MAH yoh
June	junio	HOO nyoh
July	julio	HOO lyoh
August	agosto	ah GOHS toh
September	se(p)tiembre	seh TYEHM breh (silent P)
October	octubre	ohk TOO vreh
November	noviembre	noh VYEHM breh
December	diciembre	dee SYEHM breh

winter	el invierno	ehl eem BYEHR noh
spring	la primavera	la pree mah VEH rah
summer	el verano	ehl veh RAH noh
autumn	el otoño	el oh TOH nyoh

In all cases, use *en* with these words to indicate "in," "this," "next," "last," or "every," followed (in the case of the seasons) by *el* or *la*. The context will make your meaning clear:

> I got sick last winter.
> Me enfermé en el invierno.
> meh_ehn fehr MEH_ehn ehl een BYEHR noh

> I will get sick next winter.
> Me enfermaré en el invierno.
> meh_ehn fehr mah REH ehn ehl een BYEHR noh

Numbers

0	cero	SEHR oh	6	seis	sehys
1	uno	OO noh	7	siete	SYEH teh
2	dos	dohs	8	ocho	OH choh
3	tres	trehs	9	nueve	NWEH veh
4	cuatro	KWAH troh	10	diez	dyehs
5	cinco	SEEN koh			

continues

Numbers (continued)

11	once	OHN seh	16	dieciséis	dyeh see SEHYS
12	doce	DOH seh	17	diecisiete	dyeh see SYEH teh
13	trece	TREH seh	18	dieciocho	dyeh SYOH choh
14	catorce	kah TOHR seh	19	diecinueve	dyeh see NWEH veh
15	quince	KEEN seh	20	veinte	BEYN teh

¡Ojo!

Except for 11, whenever the number 1 precedes a masculine noun, *uno* shortens to *un*, and before a feminine noun it changes to *una: veintiún años* (21 years), *veintiuna píldoras* (21 pills).

21	veintiuno	beyn TYOO noh
22	veintidós	beyn tee DOHS
30	treinta	TREYN tah
31	treinta y uno	treyn tay YOO noh
40	cuarenta	kwah REHN tah
50	cincuenta	seen KWEHN tah
60	sesenta	seh SEHN tah
70	setenta	seh TEHN tah
80	ochenta	oh CHEHN tah
90	noventa	noh VEHN tah
100	cien	syehn

(This shortened form is for exactly 100; otherwise say: ciento SYEHN toh.)

101	ciento uno	SYEHN toh_OO noh
155	ciento cincuenta y cinco	SYEHN toh seen KWEHN tay SEEN koh
200	doscientos	doh SYEHN tohs
300	trescientos	trehs SYEHN tohs
400	cuatrocientos	kwah troh SYEHN tohs
500	quinientos	kee NYEHN tohs
600	seiscientos	sey SYEHN tohs
700	setecientos	seh teh SYEHN tohs
800	ochocientos	oh choh SYEHN tohs
900	novecientos	noh veh SYEHN tohs
1,000	mil	meel
1983	mil novecientos ochenta y tres	meel noh veh SYEHN tohs oh CHEHN tay trehs
2004	dos mil cuatro	dohs meel KWAH troh

¡Ojo!

Never say y, "and," between the 100s and the 10s. Its place is between the 10s and the 1s, starting with 16 (*dieciséis*), and skipping exact multiples of 10. And remember to link it with the preceding vowel:

234 pounds
doscientos treinta y cuatro libras
doh SYEHN tohs TREHYN tay KWAH troh LEE vrahs

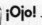

¡Ojo!

Spanish never treats thousands as multiple hundreds. Spanish speakers don't say twenty-five hundred dollars; they say two thousand five hundred dollars (in Spanish, of course).

Expressing numerical order:

Ordinal Numbers: First Things First

1st	primero	pree MEH roh (Drop or change the *O* as for *uno*.)
2nd	segundo	seh GOON doh
3rd	tercero	tehr SEH roh (Drop or change the *O* as for *uno*.)
4th	cuarto	KWAHR toh (Don't confuse with *cuatro*.)
5th	quinto	KEEN toh
6th	sexto	SEHS toh
7th	sé(p)timo	SEH tee moh (silent *P*)
8th	octavo	ohk TAH voh
9th	noveno	noh VEH noh
10th	décimo	DEH see moh

¡Ojo!

Spanish ordinals don't go any higher than 10th. A patient who lives on the 15th floor of a high-rise will say the following:

Vivo en el piso quince.
BEE voh_eh nehl PEE soh KEEN seh

Relative Quantities

more (… than)
más (… que)
mahs (… keh)

Now I eat more.
Ahora como más.
ah_OH rah KOH moh mahs

I sleep more than before.
Duermo más que antes.
DWEHR moh mahs keh_AHN tehs

less (… than)
menos (… que)
MEH nohs (… keh)

I drink less.
Tomo menos.
TOH moh MEH nohs

I drink less than before.
Tomo menos que antes.
TOH moh MEH nohs keh_AHN tehs

as ... as
tan ... como
tahn ... KOH moh

It's as strong as before.
Está tan fuerte como antes.
ehs TAH tahn FWEHR teh KOH moh_AHN tehs

as much/many as
tanto(s) como
TAHN toh(s) KOH moh

I have as many as he does.
Tengo tantos como él.
TEHN goh TAHN tohs KOH moh_ehl

so much
tanto
TAHN toh

Now he forgets so much.
Ahora él olvida tanto.
ah OH rah_ehl ohl VEE thah TAHN toh

Dates

English speakers refer to dates using ordinals (January 2nd, the 24th), but Spanish speakers use the ordinal *primero* for the first of the month only. They express all other dates using cardinal numbers (2, 15, 28, etc.). The order is day-date-month:

> Your appointment is on Tuesday, April 24th.
> Su cita es el martes, veinticuatro de abril.
> soo SEE tah_ehs ehl MAHR tehs behyn tee KWAH troh theh_ah VREEL

May 1st falls on Monday.
El primero de mayo es un lunes.
ehl pree MEHR oh deh MAH yoh_ehs oon
LOO nehs

Time

La with *una*, and *las* with the other hours, tells you
this is an "o'clock" number. To give the current
time, say the following:

What time is it?	¿Qué hora es?	keh_OH rah_ehs
It's 1:00.	Es la una.	ehs lah_OO nah
It's 2:00.	Son las dos.	sohn lahs dohs
2:15.	Las dos y cuarto.	sohn lahs dohs KWAHR toh
2:30.	Las dos y media.	sohn lahs dohs MEH thyah

Now see what happens beyond the half hour:

2:40.	Son las tres menos veinte.	sohn lahs trehs MEH nohs BEYN teh

Note that when the minutes go beyond the half
hour, Spanish speakers usually give the time using
the *next* hour *minus* the minutes, a bit like saying
"twenty to three" instead of "two forty." In the
examples shown, the first form listed is the most
common.

¡Ojo!

To say "at" a given time, don't forget the important word *a*. It's a small word that makes a big difference. Compare:

Es a la una.
ehs ah lah_OO nah
It (your appointment) is at 1:00.

Es la una.
ehs lah_OO nah
It is 1:00 (right now).

Be sure to use it in the question, too!

(At) What time is your appointment?
¿A qué hora es su cita?
ah keh_OH rah_ehs soo SEE tah

In the morning, afternoon, evening:

	With the Hour	Without the Hour
A.M./in the morning	de la mañana	por la mañana
P.M./afternoon/ evening	de la tarde	por la tarde
at night	de la noche	por la noche

Do it at 10:00 A.M.
Hágalo a las diez de la mañana.
AH gah loh_ah lahs dyehs theh lah mah NYAH nah

Do it in the morning.
Hágalo por la mañana.
AH gah loh pohr lah mah NYAH nah

Relative times:

a long time ago (with past tense verb)	hace mucho	AH seh MOO choh
already	ya	yah
before, previously, earlier	antes	AHN tehs
early	temprano	tehm PRAH noh
first	primero	pree MEH roh
for a long time (with present tense verb)	hace mucho	AH seh MOO choh
late	tarde	TAHR theh
recently	hace poco	AH seh POH koh
soon, right away	pronto	PROHN toh
then (finally)	entonces	ehn TOHN sehs
then (in a sequence)	luego	LWEH goh
then, subsequently, after(ward), later	después	dehs PWEHS

¡Ojo!

When explaining the steps of a procedure, the sequence is *primero*, then *luego* as many times as needed, and *entonces* for the last step.

More Words for Time

day	el día	ehl THEE ah
week	la semana	lah seh MAH nah
month	el mes	ehl mehs
year	el año	ehl AH nyoh

These may be followed by:

last	pasado/pasada	pah SAH thoh, pah SAH thah
next	que viene	keh BYEH neh

or preceded by:

ago	hace un/una	AH seh_OON, AH seh_OO nah
last week	la semana pasada	lah seh MAH nah pah SAH thah
next month	el mes que viene	ehl mehs keh BYEH neh
a year ago	hace un año	AH seh_oo NAH nyoh

Colors

black and blue	amoratado	ah moh rah TAH thoh
black	negro	NEH groh
blue	azul	ah SOOL
brown (complexion)	moreno	moh REH noh
brown	café	kah FEH

dark (color)	(color) oscuro	(koh LOHR) oohs KOO roh
fair (complexion)	rubio	RROO vyoh
gray	gris	gris
green	verde	BEHR theh
light (color)	(color) claro	(koh LOHR) KLAH roh
orange	anaranjado	ah nah rahn HAH thoh
pale	pálido	PAH lee thoh
pink	rosado	rroh SAH thoh
purple	morado	moh RAH thoh
red (most common and generic)	rojo	RROH hoh
white	blanco	BLAHN koh
yellow	amarillo	ah mah REE yoh

Apparel

blouse	la blusa	lah BLOO sah
coat	el abrigo	ehl ah VREE goh (heavy for weather)
coat (sport/ suit coat)	el saco	ehl SAH koh
hat	el sombrero	ehl sohm BREH roh
jacket (windbreaker or similar)	la chaqueta	lah chah KEH tah
pants (also slacks, trousers)	los pantalones	lohs pahn tah LOH nehs
shirt (dress, sport, sweat)	la camisa	lah kah MEE sah

continues

Apparel (continued)

shoes	los zapatos	lohs sah PAH tohs
socks	los calcetines	lohs kahl seh TEE nehs
stockings	las medias	lahs MEH thyahs
sweater	el suéter	ehl SWEH tehr
tee-shirt	la camiseta	lah kah mee SEH tah
underwear	la ropa interior	lah RROH pah een teh ryohr

Furniture, Equipment, and Supplies

These are some things you or your patients may refer to:

bandage	la venda	lah BEHN dah
bedpan	la chata	lah CHAH tah
blanket	la frazada	lah frah SAH thah
cabinet	el mueble	ehl MWEH vleh
cup	la taza	lah TAH sah
door	la puerta	lah PWEHR tah
drawer	el cajón	ehl kah HOHN
floor	el piso	ehl PEE soh
nightstand	la mesa de cabecera	lah MEH sah theh kah veh SEH rah
pillow	la almohada	lah ahl moh AH thah
pitcher	la jarra	lah JAH rrah
sheet	la sábana	lah SAH vah nah
shower	la ducha	lah DOO chah
sink	el lavamanos	ehl lah vah MAH nohs

soap	el jabón	ehl HAH vohn
toilet paper	el papel higiénico	ehl pah PEHL ee HYEH nee koh
toilet	el excusado	ehl ehs koo SAH thoh
towel	la toalla	lah toh AH yah
tray	la bandeja	lah bahn DEH hah
urinal	el orinal	ehl oh ree NAHL
washcloth	la toallita	lah toh ah YEE tah

The Body

ankle	el tobillo	ehl toh VEE yoh
appendix	el apéndice	ehl ah PEHN dee seh
arm	el brazo	ehl BRAH soh
armpit	la axila	lah ahk SEE lah
artery	la arteria	lah ahr TEH ryah
back	la espalda	lah ehs PAHL thah
belly (region)	el vientre	ehl BYEHN treh
bladder	la vejiga	lah beh HEE gah
blood	la sangre	lah SAHN greh
bone	el hueso	ehl WEH soh
brain	el cerebro	ehl seh REH vroh
breasts	los senos	lohs SEH nohs
buttock	la nalga	lah NAHL gah
calf	la pantorrilla	lah pahn toh RREE yah
cheek	la mejilla	lah meh HEE yah
cheekbone	el pómulo	ehl POH moo loh
chest	el pecho	ehl PEH choh

continues

The Body (continued)

chin	la barbilla	lah bahr BEE yah
collarbone	la clavícula	lah klah VEE koo lah
colon	el colon	ehl KOH lohn
diaphragm	el diafragma	ehl dyah FRAHG mah
ear	la oreja	lah oh REH hah
elbow	el codo	ehl KOH thoh
eye	el ojo	ehl OH hoh
eyebrow	la ceja	lah SEH hah
eyelash	la pestaña	lah pehs TAH nyah
eyelid	el párpado	ehl PAHR pah thoh
face	la cara	lah KAH rah
facial skin	el cutis	ehl KOO tees
finger	el dedo	ehl DEH thoh
foot	el pie	ehl pyeh
forearm	el antebrazo	ehl ahn tee BRAH soh
forehead	la frente	lah FREHN teh
gallbladder	la vesícula	lah beh SEE koo lah
genitals	los genitales	lohs heh nee TAH lehs
groin	la ingle	lah EEN gleh
gum	la encía	lah ehn SEE ah
hair (all)	el pelo	ehl PEH loh
hair (head)	el cabello	ehl kah VEH yoh
hand	la mano	lah MAH noh
head	la cabeza	lah kah VEH sah
heart	el corazón	ehl koh rah SOHN
heel	el talón	ehl tah LOHN
hip	la cadera	lah kah THEH rah
inner ear	el oído	ehl oh EE thoh
jaw	la mandíbula	lah mahn DEE boo lah

kidney	el riñón	ehl rree NYOHN
knee	la rodilla	lah rroh THEE yah
kneecap	la rótula	lah RROH too lah
large intestine	el intestino grueso	ehl een tehs TEE noh GRWEH soh
leg	la pierna	lah PYEHR nah
lip	el labio	ehl LAH vyoh
liver	el hígado	ehl EE gah thoh
lungs	los pulmones	lohs pool MOH nehs
mouth	la boca	lah BOH kah
muscle	el músculo	ehl MOOS koo loh
nail	la uña	lah OO nyah
neck	el cuello	ehl KWEH yoh
nerve	el nervio	ehl NEHR vyoh
nose	la nariz	lah nah REES
palm	la palma (de la mano)	lah PAHL mah (theh lah MAH noh)
pancreas	el páncreas	ehl PAHN kreh ahs
pelvis	la pelvis	lah PEHL vees
rectum	el recto	ehl RREHK toh
rib	la costilla	lah kohs TEE yah
shoulder	el hombro	ehl OHM broh
side	el costado	ehl kohs TAH thoh
skin	la piel	lah pyehl
small intestine	el intestino delgado	ehl een tehs TEE noh thehl gah thoh
sole	la planta (del pie)	lah PLAHN tah (thehl pyeh)
spinal column	la columna (vertebral)	lah koh LOOM nah (vehr teh brahl)

continues

The Body (continued)

spine	el espinazo	ehl ehs pee NAH soh
spleen	el bazo	ehl BAH soh
stomach	el estómago	ehl ehs TOH mah goh
temple	la sien	lah syehn
tendon	el tendón	ehl tehn DOHN
thigh	el muslo	ehl MOOS loh
throat	la garganta	lah gahr GAHN tah
toe	el dedo (del pie)	ehl DEH thoh (thehl pyeh)
tongue	la lengua	lah LEHN gwah
tonsils	las amígdalas	lahs ah MEEG dah lahs
tooth	el diente	ehl DYEHN teh
uterus	el útero	ehl OO teh roh
vein	la vena	la BEH nah
waist	la cintura	lah seen TOO rah
wrist	la muñeca	lah moo NYEH kah

Chapter 3

When the Patient Arrives

It's difficult enough to be ill or injured; add to that
seeking care from people who don't speak your language, and a simple visit to a doctor can be a fright-
ening prospect. That's why it's so important to greet
your Spanish-speaking patients in a few words they
understand. If you speak their language, even a little,
you'll put patients at ease from the start. They won't
feel constrained because they can't express themselves in English, and you'll gain better information and be able to provide better medical care.

Greeting the Patient

Unless you're dealing with an emergency, be sure
to greet the patient warmly with the polite expres-
sions and inquiries you learned in Chapter 2.

Then find out how that patient would like to communicate with you. Be careful not to assume every
Hispanic patient speaks only Spanish:

> Do you speak English?
> ¿Habla inglés?
> AH blah_een GLEHS

Would you prefer to speak English or Spanish?
¿Prefiere hablar inglés o español?
preh FYEH reh_ah BLAHR een GLEHS
oh_ehs pah NYOHL

Do you want an interpreter?
¿Desea un intérprete?
deh SEH ah_oon een TEHR preh teh

Through Their Eyes

If the patient would prefer to communicate
in Spanish, don't worry if your accent
isn't perfect or your grammar is a little
garbled. Spanish-speaking patients will be
grateful for your efforts and patient with
your shortcomings.

At the Front Desk

After the lines of communication are open, you'll
need to ask a few basic questions. Here are some
phrases you're likely to use as soon as the patient
arrives:

Can I help you?
¿En qué puedo ayudarle?
ehn keh PWEH thoh ah yoo THAHR leh

What is your name?
¿Cómo se llama Ud?
KOH moh seh YAH mah_oos TEHTH

Do you have an appointment?
¿Tiene usted una cita?
TYEH neh_oos TEHTH OO nah SEE tah

What time is your appointment?
¿Para cuándo es su cita?
PAH rah KWAHN doh_ehs soo SEE tah

Do you need an appointment now?
¿Desea sacar un turno ahora?
deh SEH ah sah KAHR TOOR noh ah OH rah

Whom are you here to see?
¿A quién deseaba ver?
ah kyehn deh she AH vah vehr

Who is your doctor?
¿Quién es su doctor?
kyehn ehs soo thohk TOHR

Is someone here with you?
¿Está usted acompañado?
ehs TAH_oos TEHTH ah kohm pah NYAH thoh

Which of you is sick?
¿Cuál de ustedes está enfermo?
kwahl theh_oos TEH thehs ehs TAH_ehn FEHR moh

Do you have a ride home?
¿Quién va a llevarle a casa?
kyehn bah_ah yeh VAHR leh_ah KAH sah

Filling Out Forms

In medicine today, forms requesting patient information are a fact of life. These phrases will help you aid your Spanish-speaking patients in filling them out:

Please fill out this form.
Favor de llenar esta planilla.
fah VOHR theh yeh NAHR EHS tah plah NEE yah

We need your permission.
Necesitamos su permiso.
neh seh see TAH mohs soo pehr MEE soh

We need your ...
Para su dirección necesitamos ...
PAH rah soo thee rehk SYOHN neh seh see TAH mohs ...

> address.
> el número de la casa.
> ehl NOO meh roh theh lah KAH sah
>
> street.
> el nombre de la calle.
> ehl NOHM breh theh lah KAH yeh

¡Ojo!

Don't waste time reinventing the wheel. Use the essential vocabulary in Chapter 2 and elsewhere to create Spanish versions of the forms you use most often.

city.
la ciudad.
lah syoo THAHTH

state.
el estado.
ehl ehs TAH thoh

zip code.
el código postal.
ehl KOH thee goh pohs TAHL

e-mail.
su dirección electrónica.
soo thee rehk SYOHN eh lehk TROH nee kah

What is your ... ?
¿Cuál es su ... ?
kwahl ehs soo

age
edad
eh THAHTH

date of birth
fecha de nacimiento
FEH chah theh nah see MYEHN toh

first language
primera lengua
pree MEH rah LEHN gwah

full name
nombre completo
NOHM breh kohm PLEH toh

first name
primer nombre
pree MEHR NOHM breh

middle initial
inicial (de segundo nombre)
ee nee SYAHL (theh seh GOON doh NOHM breh)

last name
apellido
ah peh YEE thoh

maiden name
nombre de soltera
NOHM breh theh sohl TEH rah

¡Ojo!

Spanish speakers often have two last names, the father's followed by the mother's. So in his native country, *Juan Solís Cuevas* is known as *señor Solís*, *Juan Solís Cuevas*, or *Juan Solís C.*; his *nombre* is *Juan*, his *inicial* if used is *C.* for *Cuevas*, and he is alphabetized under *S* for his father's *apellido*, *Solís*, followed by his mother's, *Cuevas*. When you help your patients, be sure they do not misinterpret the meaning of the English request for an initial.

A married woman doesn't lose her own name, but simply adds her husband's *apellido*. So if *María Soto García* marries *Juan Solís Cuevas*, she is known as *María Soto García de Solís*, or *señora María Solís* for short. However, if you ask her name or her husband introduces her, they usually give *her* name, *Soto*.

nationality
nacionalidad
nah syoh nah lee THAHTH

place of birth
lugar de nacimiento
loo GAHR theh nah see MYEHN toh

place of employment
lugar de empleo
loo GAHR theh_ehm PLEH oh

phone
teléfono
teh LEH foh noh

area code
código local
KOH thee goh loh KAHL

cell phone
(teléfono) celular móvil
seh loo LAHR MOH veel

home phone
(teléfono) residencial
reh see dehn SYAHL

pager
localizador
loh kah lee sah THOHR

work phone
(teléfono) en el trabajo
ehn ehl trah VAH hoh

race
raza
RRAH sah

relationship
parentesco
pah rehn TEHS koh

Social Security number
número de seguro social
NOO meh roh theh seh GOO roh soh
SYAHL

Do you have ... ?
¿Tiene ... ?
TYEH neh

a consent form
una (declaración de) autorización
OO nah (deh klah rah SYOHN theh) ow toh
ree sah SYOHN

a driver's license
una licencia de manejar
OO nah lee SEHN syah theh mah neh HAHR

the forms
las planillas
lahs plah NEE yahs

photo identification
prueba de identidad con foto
PRWEH vah theh_ee thehn tee THAHTH
kohn FOH toh

What's Your Occupation?

Some forms request the patient's occupation or
employment status. Here are some terms to help

fill in those blanks. (Remember to change to the
feminine *la … a* when talking with a woman.)

carpenter	el carpintero	ehl kahr peen TEH roh
cashier	el cajero	ehl kah HEH roh
clerk (office)	el funcionario	ehl foon syo NAH ryoh
cook	el cocinero	ehl koh si NEH roh
employee	el empleado	ehl ehm pleh_AH thoh
employer	empresario	ehm preh SAH ryoh
employment	empleo	ehm PLEH oh
farmer	el campesino	ehl kahm peh SEE noh
fireman	el bombero	ehl bohm BEH roh
gardener	el jardinero	ehl hahr thee NEH roh
housekeeper	el limpiador de casa	ehl leem pyah THOHR theh KAH sah
laborer	el obrero	ehl oh VREH roh
lawyer	el abogado	ehl ah voh GAH thoh
manager	el gerente	ehl heh REHN teh
mechanic	el mecánico	ehl meh KAH nee koh
nanny	la niñera	lah nee NYEH rah
painter	el pintor	ehl peen TOHR
plumber	el plomero	ehl ploh MEH roh
police officer	el policía	ehl poh lee SEE ah
priest	el cura	ehl KOO rah
salesman	el vendedor	ehl vehn deh THOHR
secretary	el secretario	ehl seh kreh TAH ryoh
student	el estudiante	ehl es too THYAHN teh
teacher	el maestro	ehl mah EHS troh
truck driver	el camionero	ehl kah myoh NEH roh
waiter	el mesero	ehl meh SEH roh

Insurance Information

A major component of any patient visit is collecting and verifying insurance information. These phrases will help you:

Do you have insurance?
¿Tiene seguro?
TYEH neh seh GHOO roh

What kind of insurance do you have?
¿Qué tipo de seguro tiene?
keh TEE poh theh seh GOO roh TYEH neh

Which is your insurance company?
¿Cuál es su aseguradora?
kwahl ehs soo_ah seh goo rah THOH rah

Can you show me your card?
¿Me muestra la tarjeta?
meh MWEHS trah lah tahr HEH tah

What is your … ?
¿Cuál es su … ?
kwahl ehs soo …

> group number
> número de grupo
> NOO meh roh theh GROO poh
>
> policy number
> número de póliza
> NOO meh roh theh POH lee sah

Have you paid your co-pay?
¿Ha pagado su porción?
ah pah GAH thoh soo pohr SYOHN

Do you have your receipt?
¿Tiene el recibo?
TYEH neh_ehl rreh SEE voh

Is this a work-related injury?
¿Se trata de un accidente de trabajo?
seh TRAH tah theh oon ahk see THEHN teh theh
trah VAH hoh

Insurance-Speak

The following terms often crop up in discussing
medical insurance. The first three are proper names,
and though they could be translated, most Spanish
speakers do not, preferring to do their best with the
English.

Blue Cross	[Cruz Azul]	kroos ah SOOL
Blue Shield	[Escudo Azul]	ehs KOO thoh_ah SOOL
Kaiser	Kaiser	KAY sehr
HMO	HMO or Organización para el Mantenimiento de la Salud	AH cheh_EH meh_oh ohr gah nee sah SYOHN PAH rah_ehl mahn teh nee MYEHN toh theh lah sah LOOTH
PPO	PPO or Organización de Proveedores Preferentes	peh peh oh ohr gah nee sah SYOHN theh proh veh_eh THOH rehs preh feh REHN tehs
disability	incapacidad	een kah pah see THATH

continues

continued

hospital	hospital	ohs pee TAHL
special programs	programas especiales	proh GRAH mahs ehs peh SYAH lehs
state aid	ayuda estatal	ah YOO thah_ehs tah TAHL
worker's compensation	compensación laboral	kohm pehn sah SYOHN lah voh RAHL

Orienting the Patient

While patients fill out forms and wait to be seen, orient them to the office and make them comfortable with the following phrases:

Make yourself comfortable.
Acomódese.
ah koh MOH theh seh

Have a seat.
Tome asiento.
TOH meh ah SYEHN toh

The bathroom is ...
El baño está ...
ehl VAH nyoh ehs TAH

> You may wait ...
> Puede esperar ...
> PWEH theh_eh speh RAHR

here	aquí	ah KEE
there	allí	ah YEE
over there	allá	ah YAH

I'm sorry, the doctor has been delayed.
Perdone, el médico se atrasa un poco.
pehr THOH neh, ehl MEH thee koh seh ah TRAH
sah oon POH koh

The doctor will see you soon.
Ya viene el médico.
yah VYEH neh_ehl MEH thee koh

Please come with me.
Favor de acompañarme.
fah VOHR theh_ah kohm pah NYAHR meh

Go with the nurse.
Acompañe a la enfermera.
ah kohm PAH nyeh_ah lah_ehn fehr MEH rah

Please see …
Por favor, diríjase a …
pohr fah VOHR dee REE hah seh …

   the nurse.
   la enfermera.
   lah ehn fehr MEH rah

   the receptionist.
   la recepcionista.
   lah reh sehp syoh NEES tah

   the secretary.
   la secretaria.
   lah seh kreh TAH ryah

Past the Waiting Room

After registration is complete, and before the doctor
sees the patient, a nurse or other assistant often

briefly interviews the patient and gathers some basic physical information. The following words and phrases, plus the essential queries in Chapter 2, will help you in these tasks.

Vital Statistics

Please step on the scale.
Suba a la báscula.
SOO vah_ah la VAHS koo lah

Please remove your shoes.
¿Se quita los zapatos?
seh KEE TAH lohs sah PAH tohs

Please stand as tall as possible.
Yérgase lo más posible.
YEHR gah seh loh mahs poh SEE vleh

I need to take your blood pressure.
Necesito tomarle la presión.
neh seh SEE toh toh MAHR leh lah preh SYOHN

Please roll up your sleeve.
¿Se arremanga, por favor?
seh ah rreh MAHN gah pohr fah VOHR

I need to take your temperature.
Vamos a ver su temperatura.
BAH mohs ah vehr soo tehm peh rah TOO rah

Please hold the thermometer under your tongue.
El termómetro debe estar debajo de la lengua.
ehl tehr MOH meh troh THEH veh_ehs TAHR
theh VAH hoh thed lah LEHN gwah

Please hold still for just a moment.
Favor de no moverse por un momento.
fah VOHR theh noh moh VEHR seh pohr oon moh
MEHN toh

We will need a urine specimen.
Necesitamos un espécimen de su orina.
neh seh see TAH mohs oon ehs PEH see mehn theh
soo_oh REE nah

Please use this cup.
Orine directamente en esta vasija.
oh REE neh thee rehk tah MEHN teh_ehn EHS
tah vah SEE hah

Cover it to prevent contamination.
Tápela para que no se contamine.
TAH peh lah PAH rah keh noh seh kohn tah
MEE neh

Bring it out to me when you are ready.
Favor de traérmelo cuando haya terminado.
fah VOHR theh trah HER meh loh KWAN
doh_AH yah tehr mee NAH thoh

You may leave the sample in there.
Puede dejar la muestra allí dentro.
PWEH theh deh HAHR lah MWEHS trah_ah
YEE THEHN troh

Medications, Reactions

Are you currently taking any medications?
¿Toma actualmente algunos medicamentos?
TOH mah ahk twal MEHN teh_ahl GOO nohs
meh thee kah MEHN tohs

What are they?

¿Cuáles son?

KWAH lehs sohn

Are you allergic to any medications?

¿Es alérgico a algún medicamento?

ehs ah LEHR hee koh_ah_ahl GOON meh thee kah MEHN toh

Which (ones)?

¿Cuál? ¿Cuáles?

kwahl KWAH lehs

Current Issue

What brings you in today?

¿Por qué ha venido a vernos hoy?

pohr keh_ah veh NEE thoh_ah VEHR nohs oy

What problem are you having?

¿Qué problema le afecta?

keh proh VLEH mah leh_ah FEHK tah?

Do you have pain?

¿Le duele algo?

leh THWEH leh_ahl goh

Where does it hurt?

¿Dónde le duele?

DOHN deh leh DWEH leh

When did it start?

¿Cuándo empezó el dolor?

KWAHN doh_ehm peh SOH_ehl thoh LOHR

On a scale of 0 to 10, with 10 being the worst, what number is your pain?

Si cero significa ningún dolor y diez el peor posible, ¿en qué número califica el suyo?

see SEH roh seeg nee FEE kah neen GOON doh LOHR ee dyehs ehl peh OHR poh SEE vleh, ehn keh NOO meh roh kah lee FEE kah_ehl SOO yoh

Please remove ...
Favor de quitarse ...
fah VOHR theh kee TAHR seh ...

> all your clothing.
> toda la ropa.
> TOH thah lah RROH pah
>
> everything except your underwear.
> todo menos la ropa interior.
> TOH thoh MEH nohs lah RROH pah_een teh RYOHR
>
> everything from the waist up.
> todo desde la cintura para arriba.
> TOH thoh THEHS theh lah SEEN TOO rah PAH rah_ah RREE vah
>
> everything from the waist down.
> todo desde la cintura para abajo.
> TOH thoh THEHS theh lah seen TOO rah PAH rah_ah VAH hoh

Please put on this gown.
Póngase esta bata
POHN gah seh_EHS tah VAH tah

> with the opening …
> para que abra …
> PAH rah keh AH vrah …

>> in front.
>> por delante.
>> pohr theh LAHN teh

>> in back.
>> por detrás.
>> pohr theh TRAHS

The doctor will be in shortly.
No tardará el médico.
noh tahr thah RAH_ehl MEH thee koh

So much for the preliminaries; in the next chapter, you'll find the words and phrases to gather a detailed patient history.

Chapter 4

Taking the Medical History

A patient's medical history can be complex. Luckily, the Spanish you'll need to take it is not. The questions are formed simply, and many are structured in the same way. After you get started, you'll be surprised how easy it is to get the detailed information you need.

Who's Your *Other* Doctor?

There are times you'll see patients for whom you are not the primary-care physician. When you do, you'll want to know the following:

How has your health been up until now?
Hasta ahora, ¿Cómo ha estado de salud?
AHS tah_ah OH rah KOH moh_ah ehs TAH thoh theh sah LOOTH

Who is your doctor?
¿Quién es su doctor?
kyehn ehs soo thohk TOHR

Where can I contact him (her)?
¿Dónde puedo comunicarme con él (ella)?
DOHN deh PWEH thoh koh moo nee KAHR meh kohn ehl (EH yah)

When was the last time you visited him (her)?
¿Cuándo fue la última vez que lo (la) visitó?
KWAHN doh fweh lah_OOL tee mah vehs keh loh
(lah) vee see TOH

What was the purpose of the visit?
¿Por qué consultó con su médico?
pohr keh kohn sool TOH kohn soo MEH thee koh

Past Illnesses and Injuries and Family History

Note: For a more comprehensive list of illnesses and
conditions, see Chapter 7. For questions concerning
current symptoms and conditions, see Chapter 5.

Have you ever had …
¿Ha tenido antes …
ah teh NEE thoh_AHN tehs

Has anyone in your immediate family (parents,
grandparents, brothers, sisters) had …
Entre sus abuelos, padres, y hermanos, ¿ha
habido algún caso de …
EHN treh soos ah VWEH lohs PAH threhs
ee_ehr MAH nohs ah_ah VEE thoh_ahl
GOON KAH soh theh

bronchitis?	bronquitis?	brohn KEE tees
cancer?	cáncer?	KAHN sehr/keh
What type?	¿Qué tipo?	TEE poh
cerebral infarct/ stroke?	derrame cerebral?	deh RRAH meh she reh VRAHL
convulsions?	convulsiones?	kohn bool SYOH nehs

diabetes?	diabetes?	dyah VEH tehs
glaucoma?	glaucoma?	glaw KOH mah
heart disease?	enfermedad del corazón?	ehn fehr meh THAHTH thehl koh rah SOHN
high blood pressure?	presión alta?	preh SYOHN AHL tah
high cholesterol?	colesterol elevado?	koh lehs teh ROHL eh leh VAH thoh
kidney disease?	enfermedad de los ríones?	ehn fehr meh THAHTH tehh lohs ree NYOH nehs
low blood pressure?	presión baja?	preh SYOHN BAH hah
pneumonia?	pulmonía?	pool moh NEE ah
psychiatric problems?	problemas emocionales?	proh VLEH mahs eh moh syoh NAH lehs
respiratory problems?	problemas respiratorios?	proh VLEH mahs rrehs pee rah TOH ryohs
thrombo-phlebitis/ blood clots?	tromboflebitis?	trohm boh fleh VEE tees
tuberculosis?	tuberculosis?	too vehr koo LOH sees
venereal diseases?	enfermedades venéreas?	ehn fehr meh THAH thehs veh NEH reh ahs
AIDS?	SIDA?	SEE thah

Have you had any other diseases?
¿Ha padecido de cualquier otra enfermedad?
ah pah theh SEE thoh theh kwahl KYEHR OH
trah_ehn fehr meh THAHTH

Which?
¿Cuál?
kwahl

Are your parents/grandparents living?
¿Todavía viven sus padres/abuelos?
toh thah VEE ah VEE vehn soos PAH threhs/ah VWEH lohs

Are your brothers/sisters living?
¿Todavía viven sus hermanos?
toh thah VEE ah VEE vehn soos ehr MAH nohs

What did your [family member] die of?
¿De qué murió su [family member]?
deh keh moo RYOH soo

Have you ever been hit in the ...
¿Se ha golpeado ...
seh_ah gohl peh_AH thoh

head?	la cabeza?	lah kah VEH sah
face?	la cara?	lah KAH rah
neck?	el cuello?	ehl KWEH yoh
eyes?	los ojos?	lohs OH hohs
ears?	los oídos?	lohs oh EE thohs
nose?	la nariz?	lah nah REES

Have you ever lost consciousness?
¿Ha perdido el conocimiento?
ah pehr THEE thoh_ehl koh noh see MYEHN toh

For how long?
¿Por cuánto tiempo?
pohr KWAHN toh TYEHM poh

When?
¿Cuándo?
KWAHN doh

What happened?
¿Qué le pasó?
keh leh pah SOH

Is there anything else you would like to tell me?
¿Hay algo más que quiera decirme?
ay AHL goh mahs keh KYEH rah theh SEER meh

Allergies

Are you allergic to ...
¿Tiene alergia a ...
TYEH neh_ah LEHR hyah_ah

any foods?	alguna comida?	ahl GOO nah koh MEE thah
eggs?	los huevos?	lohs WEH vohs
milk?	la leche?	lah leh cheh
dairy products?	los productos lácteos?	lohs proh THOOK tohs LAHK teh ohs
seafood?	los mariscos?	lohs mah REES kohs
other?	cualquier otra?	kwahl KYEHR OH trah
any medicines?	alguna medicina?	ahl GOO nah meh thee SEE nah
aspirin?	la aspirina?	lah_ahs pee REE nah
penicillin?	la penicilina?	lah peh nee see LEE nah
sulfa?	la sulfa?	lah SOOL FAH

continues

continued

other antibiotics?	otros antibióticos?	OH trohs ahn tee BYOH tee kohs
iodine?	el yodo?	ehl YOH thoh
contrast medium?	medio de contraste?	MEH thyoh theh kohn TRAHS teh
dust?	el polvo?	ehl POHL voh
grass?	la grama?	lah GRAH mah
insect bites?	las picaduras de insecto?	lahs pee kah THOO rahs theh_een SEHK toh
poison ivy?	la hiedra venenosa?	lah YEH thrah veh neh NOH sah
poison oak?	la encina venonosa?	lah_ehn SEE nah veh neh NOH sah
pollen?	el polen?	ehl POH lehn
animals?	los animales?	lohs ah nee MAH lehs

When asking about animal allergies (or bites), use the words in the following table to identify the culprit.

Note: Different Spanish speakers may use different words for the same animal. Where you see options below, use them to find the term familiar to your patient.

When Animals Strike Back

ant	la hormiga	lah_ohr MEE gah
bee	la abeja	lah_ah VEH hah
bird	el pájaro	ehl PAH hah roh
cat	el gato	ehl GAH toh
dog	el perro	ehl PEH rroh
mosquito	el mosquito	ehl mohs KEE toh
	el zancudo	ehl sahn KOO thoh

mouse	el ratón	ehl rrah TOHN
rat	la rata	lah RRAH tah
scorpion	el escorpión	ehl ehs kohr PYOHN
	el alacrán	ehl ah lah KRAHN
snake	la víbora	lah VEE voh rah
	la culebra	lah koo LEH vrah
	la serpiente	lah sehr PYEHN teh
spider	la araña	lah ah RAH nyah
squirrel	la ardilla	lah ahr THEE yah

What is the allergic reaction like?

¿Cómo es la reacción alérgica?

KOH moh_ehs lah rreh ahk SYOHN ah LEHR hee kah

Do you get …

¿Reacciona con …

reh ahk SYOH nah kohn

rash?	una erupción?	OO nah_eh roop SYOHN
shortness of breath?	una falta de aire?	OO nah FAHL tah theh_AY reh
swelling?	una hinchazón?	OO nah_een chah SOHN

Past Surgeries and Hospitalizations

Have you ever been in the hospital?

¿Ha estado alguna vez en el hospital?

ah_ehs TAH thoh_ahl GOO nah vehs ehn ehl ohs pee TAHL

Why were you there?
¿Por qué?
pohr keh

When was it?
¿Cuándo fue?
KWAHN doh fweh

How long were you there?
¿Cuánto tiempo estuvo allí?
KWAHN toh TYEHM poh_ehs TOO voh_ah YEE

Have you ever had surgery?
¿Ha sido operado alguna vez?
ah SEE thoh_oh peh RAH thoh_ahl GOO nah vehs

What was the surgery for?
¿Para qué fue?
PAH rah keh fweh

Immunizations and Tests

Have you had vaccinations for …
¿Le han puesto vacunas de …
leh_ahn PWEHS toh vah KOO nahs theh

cholera?	la cólera?	lah KOH leh rah
diphteria?	la difteria?	lah theef TEH ryah
hepatitis A or B?	la hepatitis A o B?	lah eh pah TEE tees ah oh veh
measles?	el sarampión?	ehl sah rahm PYOHN
polio?	el polio?	ehl POH lyoh
rubella?	la rubeola?	lah roo veh_OH lah
smallpox?	la viruela?	lah bee RWEH lah
tetanus?	el tétano?	TEH tah noh

| typhoid fever? | la fiebre tifoidea? | lah FYEH vreh tee foy THEH ah |
| whooping cough? | la tos ferina? | lah tohs feh REE nah |

When?
¿Cuándo?
KWAHN doh

Have you ever had a chest x-ray?
¿Le han tomado una radiografía del pecho?
leh ahn toh MAH thoh_OO nah RRAH thyoh grah FEE ah thehl PEH choh

When and where was it taken?
¿Cuándo se la tomaron? ¿Dónde?
KWAHN doh seh lah toh MAH rohn/DOHN deh

What were the results?
¿Cuál fue el resultado?
kwahl fweh_ehl rreh sool TAH thoh

Have you had a tuberculosis test?
¿Le han hecho una prueba de tuberculosis?
leh_ahn EH choh_OO nah PRWEH vah theh too vehr koo LOH sees

Where were you tested?
¿Dónde se la dieron?
DOHN deh seh lah DYEH rohn

At what facility were you tested?
¿En qué facilidad médica le hicieron la prueba?
ehn keh fah see lee THAHTH leh_ee SYEH rohn lah PRWEH vah

Were the results positive or negative?
¿Resultó positiva o negativa la prueba?
rreh sool TOH poh see TEE vah oh neh gah TEE
vah lah PRWEH vah

Have you ever had a blood transfusion?
¿Ha recibido una transfusión de sangre?
ah rreh see VEE thoh_OO nah trahns foo
SYOHN deh SAHN greh

Travels Abroad

Have you ever traveled outside this country?
¿Ha viajado fuera de este país?
ah vyah HAH thoh FWEH rah theh_EHS teh
pah EES

When?
¿Cuándo?
KWAHN doh

Where?
¿A dónde?
ah THOHN deh

Were you sick?
¿Se enfermó?
seh_ehn fehr MOH

Did you see a doctor while in that country?
¿Vio a un médico allá?
byoh_ah_oon MEH thee koh_ah YAH

What was the diagnosis?
¿Cuál fue su diagnosis?
kwahl fweh soo thyahg NOH sees

What treatment did you receive?
¿Qué tratamiento le dio?
keh trah tah MYEHN toh leh dyoh

Have you had any more problems with this illness
since the first time?
Desde entonces, ¿ha vuelto a tener problemas con
esta enfermedad?
DEHS theh_ehn TOHN sehs ah VWEHL toh_ah
teh NEHR proh VLEH mahs kohn EHS tah_ehn
fehr meh THAHTH

Social Habits

Do you sleep well?
¿Duerme bien?
DWEHR meh vyehn

How is your appetite?
¿Cómo está su apetito?
KOH moh_ehs TAH soo_ah peh TEE toh

Has your weight changed recently?
¿Ha subido o bajado de peso últimamente?
ah soo VEE thoh_oh vah HAH thoh theh PEH
soh_OOL tee mah mehn teh

Do you drink coffee?
¿Bebe/¿Toma cafe?
BEH veh/TOH mah kah FEH

Do you drink tea?
¿Bebe/¿Toma té?
BEH veh/TOH mah teh

How many cups a day?
¿Cuántas tazas cada día?
KWAHN tahs TAH sahs KAH thah THEE ah

Smoking

Do you smoke/use ...
¿Fuma/¿Usa ...
FOO mah/OO sah

cigarettes?	cigarrillos?	see gah RREE yohs
pipe?	pipa?	PEE pah
cigars?	cigarros?	see GAH rrohs
chewing tobacco?	rapé?	rrah PEH
marijuana?	marihuana?	mah ree WAH nah

How much do you smoke a day?
¿Cuánto fuma al día?
KWAHN toh FOO mah ahl THEE ah

How long have you been smoking?
¿Cuánto hace que fuma?
KWAHN toh_AH seh keh FOO mah

How long ago did you stop smoking?
¿Cuánto hace que no fuma?
KWAHN toh_AH seh keh noh FOO mah

Have you tried to stop smoking?
¿Ha tratado de dejar de fumar?
ah trah TAH thoh theh theh HAR theh foo MAR

Would you like to stop smoking?
¿Le gustaría dejar de fumar?
leh goos tah REE ah theh HAHR theh foo MAHR

Alcohol Use

Do you drink …
¿Bebe …/¿Toma …
BEH veh/ TOH mah

beer?	cerveza?	sehr VEH sah
brandy?	aguardiente?	ah gwahr DYEHN teh
liquor?	bebidas fuertes?	beh VEE thahs FWEHR tehs
wine?	vino?	BEE noh

How many glasses a day?
¿Cuántos vasos cada día?
KWAHN tohs VAH sohs KAH thah THEE ah

Alcohol Abuse

To discover whether your patient has a serious
drinking problem:

Do you have to drink more or less to get drunk than
you used to?
Últimamente, ¿tiene que tomar más o menos que
antes para emborracharse?
OOL tee mah MEHN teh, TYEH neh keh toh
MAHR mahs oh MEH nohs keh_AHN tehs PAH
rah_ehm boh rrah CHAHR seh

Do you get drunk when you don't mean to?
¿Se emborracha sin querer?
seh_ehm boh RRAH chah seen keh REHR

Do you eat food when you drink, or do you forget to eat?
¿Come cuando toma, o se le olvida comer?
KOH meh KWAHN doh TOH mah, oh seh leh_ohl VEE thah koh MEHR

Do you ever see things that are not there?
¿A veces ve cosas que no están allí?
ah VEH sehs veh KOH sahs keh noh_ehs TAHN ah YEE

How much time do you spend ...
¿Cuánto tiempo pasa ...
KWAHN toh TYEHM poh PAH sah

> drinking?
> tomando (alcohol)?
> toh MAHN doh_ahl koh OHL
>
> thinking about drinking?
> pensando en tomar?
> pehn SAHN doh_ehn toh MAHR
>
> recovering from drinking episodes?
> recuperándose de una borrrachera?
> rreh koo peh RAHN doh seh theh_OO nah voh rrah CHEH rah

When you stop drinking, do you have ...
Cuando deja de tomar alcohol, ¿tiene ...
KWAHN doh THEH hah theh toh MAHR ahl koh OHL, TYEH neh

> difficulty sleeping?
> dificultad para dormir?
> thee fee kool TAHTH PAH rah thohr MEER

nausea?
náuseas?
NOW seh ahs

nervousness?
agitación?
ah hee tah SYOHN

sweating?
sudores?
soo THOH rehs

tremors?
temblores?
tehm BLOH rehs

vomiting?
vómitos?
VOH mee tohs

Do you drink to stop any of these symptoms?
¿Toma para aliviar estos síntomas?
TOH mah PAH rah_ah lee VYAHR EHS tohs
SEEN toh mahs

Have you ever had …
¿Ha sufrido de …
ah soo FREE thoh theh

blackouts?
lapsos de conocimiento?
LAHP sohs theh koh noh see MYEHN toh

hangovers?
resacas?
rreh SAH kahs

Has anyone ever told you that you have a drinking problem?

¿Le ha indicado otra persona que usted tiene problema con la bebida alcohólica?

leh_ah_een dee KAH thoh_OH trah pehr SOH nah keh_oos TEHTH TYEH neh proh VLEH mah kohn lah veh VEE thah ahl koh OH lee kah

Would you like help?

¿Quiere ayuda?

KYEH reh_ah YOO thah

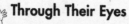 **Through Their Eyes**

Many Spanish speakers simply do not think of beer and wine as "alcohol consumption." Beer is a refreshing *bebida* (drink), and wine is part of a *comida* (meal). Make your questions explicit: How much beer do you drink? *¿Cuánta cerveza toma?*

Drug Abuse

When you know or suspect your patient is using drugs inappropriately, these phrases will help you discover the facts:

Do you use any drugs or prescription medicines?

¿Usa drogas o medicinas recetadas?

OO sah throh gahs oh meh thee SEE nahs rreh seh TAH thahs

Which ones?

¿Cuáles?

KWAH lehs

Why do you use them?
¿Por qué las usa?
pohr keh lahs OO sah

How long have you used them?
¿Cuánto tiempo hace que las usa?
KWAHN toh TYEHM poh_AH seh keh lahs OO sah

Have you ever shared needles?
¿Ha compartido agujas?
ah kohm pahr TEE thoh_ah GOO hahs

Have you ever shared needles with someone with ...
¿Ha compartido agujas con alguien que tenga ...
ah kohm pahr TEE thoh_ah GOO hahs kohn AHL
gyehn keh TEHN gah

| hepatitis? | hepatitis? | eh pah TEE tees |
| AIDS? | SIDA? | SEE thah |

Do you think you have a drug use problem?
¿Cree que abusa de las drogas?
KREH eh keh_ah VOO sah theh lahs THROH gahs

Would you like help?
¿Quiere ayuda?
KYEH reh_ah YOO thah

Chapter 5

The Physical Exam

A physical exam provides vital information, but it also means giving commands, touching the patient, and invading his or her personal space.

To soften the commands, use the polite forms shown in Chapter 2. And with Hispanic patients, proximity and physical contact can be positives. For Spanish speakers, standing close is the norm, and touching is an acceptable part of body language. You actually improve communication by offering an arm when you ask the patient to sit or lie down, or when you stand nearby and guide the patient's actions.

Such gestures will gain your patient's trust and offset any small errors you might make in grammar or pronunciation.

What Brings You In?

At the start of any physical exam, the most important question is usually this:

> What problem brings you here today?
> ¿Qué problema ha provocado esta visita?
> keh proh VLEH mah_ah proh voh KAH thoh
> EHS tah vee SEE tah

The answer is likely to be one of the following:

allergies	alergias	ah LEHR hyahs
backache	dolor de espalda	doh LOHR theh_ehs PAHL thah
bleeding	sangramiento	sahn grah MYEHN tohs
bloody bowel movement	sangre en las heces	SAHN greh_ehn lahs EH sehs
bloody urine	sangre en la orina	SAHN greh_ehn lah_oh REE nah
breathing difficulty	la respiración penosa	lah rrehs pee rah SYOHN peh NOH sah
chest pain	dolor en el pecho	doh LOHR ehn ehl PEH choh
chills	escalofríos	ehs kah loh FREE ohs
coughing	tos	tohs
coughing blood	tos con sangre	tohs kohn SAHN greh
depression	depresión	deh preh SYOHN
diarrhea	diarrea	dyah RREH ah
fever	fiebre	FYEH vreh
gas (upper)	gas	gahs
gas (lower)	flato	FLAH toh
headache	dolor de cabeza	doh LOHR theh kah VEH sah
hemorrhoids (popular)	almorranas	ahl moh RRAH nahs
indigestion	indigestión	een dee hehs TYOHN

nausea	náusea	NOW seh ah
numbness/ tingling	entumecimiento/ anquilosamiento	ehn too meh see MYEHN toh/ahn kee loh sah MYEHN toh
palpitations	palpitaciones	pahl pee tah SYOH nehs
severe pain	dolores fuertes	doh LOH rehs FWEHR tehs
sexually transmitted disease	enfermedad transmitida sexualmente	ehn fehr meh THAHTH trahns mee TEE thah sehk swahl MEHN teh
skin problems	problemas con la piel	proh VLEH mahs kohn lah pyehl
slurred speech	el habla mascullada	ehl AH vlah mahs koo YAH thah
sore throat	dolor de garganta	doh LOHR theh gahr GAHN tah
vaginal discharge	descarga vaginal	dehs KAHR gah vah HEE nahl
visual problems	problemas con la vista	proh VLEH mahs kohn lah VEES tah
vomiting	vómitos	BOH mee tohs
vomiting blood	sangre en el vómito	SAHN greh_ehn ehl BOH mee toh
weight gain (unexplained)	un aumento de peso (inexplicado)	oon ow MEHN toh theh PEH soh_een ehks plee KAH thoh
weight loss (unexplained)	una pérdida de peso (inexplicada)	OO nah PEHR thee thah theh PEH soh_ een ehks plee KAH thah

You'll find more Spanish names of symptoms, illnesses, and conditions in other chapters of this guide.

Say "Ah"

Once you know the problem, these phrases will help you find its source:

I am going to …
Voy a …
boy ah

> examine you. (male)
> examinarlo.
> ehk sah mee NAHR loh

> examine you. (female)
> examinarla.
> ehk sah mee NAHR lah

>> take your …
>> tomarle …
>> toh MAHR leh

>>> temperature.
>>> la temperatura.
>>> lah tehm peh rah TOO rah

>>> pulse.
>>> el pulso.
>>> ehl POOL soh

>>> blood pressure.
>>> la presión arterial.
>>> lah preh SYOHN ahr teh RYAHL

>>> listen to your chest.
>>> auscultarle el pecho.
>>> ows kool TAHR leh_ehl PEH choh

Please …
Por favor …
pohr fah VOHR

> take a deep, slow breath.
> respire despacio y profundo.
> rrehs PEE reh thehs PAH syoh_ee proh
> FOON doh

> now breathe normally.
> ahora respire normalmente.
> ah_OH rah rrehs PEE reh nohr mahl MEHN
> teh

> stand up straight and close your eyes.
> yérgase y cierre los ojos.
> YEHR gah seh_ee SYEH rreh lohs OH hohs

> walk one foot in front of the other.
> camine poniendo un pie delante del otro.
> kah MEE neh poh NYEHN doh_oon pyeh
> theh LAHN teh thehl OH troh

> push on my hands.
> empuje contra mis manos.
> ehm POO heh KOHN trah mees MAH nohs

> pull my hands.
> tire de mis manos.
> TEE reh theh mees MAH nohs

> bend over …
> inclínese …
> een KLEE neh seh

> sit down.
> siéntese.
> SYEHN teh seh

stand up.
levántese.
leh VAHN teh seh

lie down.
acuéstese en su ..../échese en su ....
ah KWEHS teh seh_ehn soo/EH cheh
seh_ehn soo

lie still.
quédese quieto.
KEH theh seh KYEH toh

turn over.
dése vuelta.
DEH seh VWEHL tah

turn your head.
vuelva la cabeza.
BWEHL vah lah kah VEH sah

do that again.
vuelva a hacer eso otra vez.
BWEHL vah_ah_ah SEHR EH soh_OH trah
vehs

You need more tests.
Necesita más pruebas.
neh seh SEE tah mahs PRWEH vahs

When we have the results, we'll know more.
Sabremos más cuando tengamos los resultados.
sah VREH mohs mahs KWAHN doh tehn GAH
mohs lohs rreh sool TAH thohs

Words of Comfort

Let's face it. Some examinations can be unpleasant for the patient. To acknowledge that and offer reassurance, use these phrases:

Are you comfortable?
¿Está cómodo?
ehs TAH KOH moh thoh

This won't hurt.
Esto no le dolerá.
EHS toh noh leh doh leh RAH

You may get dressed now.
Puede vestirse ahora.
PWEH theh vehs TEER seh_ah OH rah

I'll be back in a minute to talk to you.
Volveré dentro de un minuto para hablar con usted.
bohl veh REH DEHN troh deh_oon mee NOO
toh PAH rah_ah VLAHR kohn oos TEHTH

Abuse and Assault

If you know a patient has been assaulted or you suspect abuse, you'll need to ask some straightforward questions. Victims of abuse often feel they in some way deserve it, or lie about the source of their injuries, so you must phrase your questions carefully. It's often helpful to ask about the sequence of events, rather than the reasons for them:

What were you doing when this happened?
¿Qué hacía cuando esto ocurrió?
keh_ah SEE ah KWAHN doh_EHS toh_oh koo
RRYOH

Did someone do this to you on purpose?
¿Alguien le hizo esto adrede?
AHL gyehn leh_EE soh_EHS toh_ah THREH theh

Were you raped?
¿La violó?
lah vyoh LOH

A specialist will handle the examination.
Un especialista se encargará del examen.
oon ehs peh syah LEES tah seh_ehn kahr gah RAH
thehl ehk SAH mehn

Don't be afraid to tell me everything.
No tenga miedo de decírmelo todo.
Noh TEHN gah MYEH thoh theh theh SEER
meh loh TOH thoh

I have to notify the authorities.
Tengo que notificar a las autoridades.
TEHN goh keh noh tee fee KAHR ah lahs ow toh
ree THAH thehs

Pain

To identify and locate pain, use these phrases. If
what hurts the patient is plural, *duele* becomes *duelen:* Does your foot hurt? *¿Le duele el pie?*; Do your
feet hurt? *¿Le duelen los pies?*

Do you have pain?
¿Le duele algo?
leh DWEH leh_AHL goh

Where does it hurt?
¿Dónde le duele?
DOHN deh leh DWEH leh

When did it start?
¿Cuándo empezó el dolor?
KWAHN doh_ehm peh SOH_ehl thoh LOHR

Is this the first time you have had this type of pain?
¿Es la primera vez que ha tenido este tipo de dolor?
ehs lah pree MEH rah vehs keh_ah teh NEE
thoh_ehs teh TEE poh theh thoh LOHR

When was the first time?
¿Cuándo fue la primera vez?
KWAHN doh fweh lah pree MEH rah vehs

How long does the pain last each time?
¿Cuánto duró el dolor cada vez?
KWAHN toh thoo ROH_ehl thoh LOHR kah
thah vehs

On a scale of 0 to 10, with 10 being the worst, what
number is your pain?
Si cero significa ningún dolor y diez el peor posible, ¿qué número le pone al suyo?
see SEH roh seeg nee FEE kah neen GOON doh
LOHR ee dyehs ehl mah YOHR poh SEE vleh,
keh NOO meh roh leh POH neh_ahl SOO yoh

Did it begin ...
¿Comenzó ...
koh mehn SOH

    slowly?
    lentamente?
    lehn tah MEHN teh

    suddenly?
    de repente?
    deh rreh PEHN teh

Can you describe the pain?
¿Puede describir el dolor?
PWEH theh thehs kree VEER ehl thoh LOHR

> Is the pain ...
> ¿Es un dolor ...
> ehs oon doh LOHR ...

Types of Pain

dull?	sordo?	SOHR thoh
sharp?	agudo?	ah GOO thoh
constant?	constante?	kohn STAHN teh
intermittent?	intermitente?	een tehr mee TEHN teh
mild?	leve?	LEH veh
moderate?	moderado?	moh theh RAH thoh
severe?	severo?	seh VEH roh
pressurelike?	opresivo?	oh preh SEE voh
burning?	quemante?	keh MAHN teh
cramping?	acalambrado?	ah kah lahm BRAH thoh

Does the pain move?
¿Se cunde el dolor?
seh KOON deh_ehl thoh LOHR

From where to where?
¿Hacia dónde?
AH syah THOHN deh

Is the pain stronger (weaker)?
¿El dolor es más fuerte (menos fuerte)?
ehl thoh LOHR ehs mahs FWEHR teh_oh MEH
nohs FWEHR the

Where does it hurt …
¿Dónde le duele …
DOHN deh leh DWEH leh

> the most?
> más?
> mahs
>
> the least?
> menos?
> MEH nohs

Do you have the pain …
¿Tiene dolor …
TYEH neh thoh LOHR

When Does It Hurt?

all the time?	todo el tiempo?	TOH thoh_ehl TYEHM poh
in the morning?	por la mañana?	pohr lah mah NYAH nah
in the afternoon/ evening?	por la tarde?	pohr lah TAHR theh
at night?	por la noche?	pohr lah NOH cheh
before eating?	antes de comer?	AHN tehs theh koh MEHR
while eating?	mientras come?	MYEHN trahs KOH meh
after eating?	después de comer?	dehs PWEHS theh koh MEHR

Do you have the pain ...
¿Tiene dolor ...
TYEH neh thoh LOHR

> when you ...
> cuando usted ...
> KWAHN doh_oos TEHTH

are upset?	está trastornado?	ehs TAH trahs tohr NAH thoh
bend over?	se inclina?	seh_een KLEE nah
climb stairs?	sube escaleras?	SOO veh ehs kah LEH RAHS
defecate?	evacúa el vientre?	eh vah KOO_ah ehl VYEHN treh
exercise?	hace ejercicio?	ah seh_eh hehr SEE syoh
have sex?	se une sexualmente?	seh_OO neh sehk swahl MEHN teh
lie down?	se echa?	seh_eh chah
stand?	se pone de pie?	seh POH neh theh pyeh
swallow?	traga?	TRAH gah
urinate?	orina?	oh REE nah
walk?	camina?	kah MEE nah

Is there any numbness?
¿Está entumecido/adormecido?
ehs TAH_ehn too meh SEE thoh/ah thohr meh SEE thoh

Is there anything that makes the pain ...
¿Hay algo que ...
ay AHL goh keh ...

better?
alivie el dolor?
ah LEE vyeh_ehl thoh LOHR

worse?
aumente el dolor?
ow MEHN teh_ehl thoh LOHR

Does the pain wake you at night?
¿Le despierta el dolor en la noche?
leh dehs PYEHR tah_ehl doh LOHR ehn lah NOH
cheh

Does the pain go away after you rest?
¿Se va el dolor después de que usted descansa?
seh vah_ehl thoh LOHR dehs PWEHS theh
keh_oos TEHTH thehs KAHN sah

Do you take anything for the pain?
¿Toma algo para el dolor?
TOH mah_ahl goh PAH rah_ehl doh LOHR

Does it help?
¿Lo alivia?
loh_ah LEE vyah

Cardiovascular and Cardiorespiratory Systems

Breathe deeply through your mouth.
Respire profundo por la boca.
rrehs PEE reh proh FOON doh pohr lah VOH kah

Breathe normally.
Respire normalmente.
rehs PEE reh nohr mahl MEHN teh

Cough.
Tosa.
TOH sah

Say "33" in English.
En inglés diga "thirty-three."
ehn een GLEHS THEE gah "thirty-three"

Say "e."
Diga "iiii."
DEE gah ee

Do you get dizzy after exertion?
¿Se marea cuando se esfuerza?
seh mah REH_ah KWAN doh seh_ehs FWEHR sah

Do you have or have you had pain in your chest?
¿Tiene ahora o ha tenido antes dolor en el pecho?
TYEH neh_ah OH rah_oh_ah teh NEE
thoh_AHN tehs doh LOHR ehn ehl PEH choh

Is it worse when you ...
¿Es peor cuando ...
ehs peh OHR KWAHN doh

> inhale?
> aspira?
> ahs PEE rah
>
> exhale?
> espira?
> ehs PEE rah
>
> exert yourself?
> se esfuerza?
> seh_ehs FWEHR sah

Do you have difficulty in breathing while …
¿Tiene dificultad con la respiración cuando está …
TYEH neh thee fee kool TAHTH kohn lah rrehs
pee rah SYOHN KWAHN doh ehs TAH

> sitting?
> sentado?
> sehn TAH thoh

> standing?
> de pie?
> theh pyeh

> lying down?
> acostado?
> ah kohs TAH thoh

> exerting yourself?
> esforzándose?
> ehs fohr SAHN doh seh

Does the problem go away when you stop?
¿Se va el problema cuando usted cesa?
seh vah_ehl proh VLEH mah KWAHN doh_oos
TEHTH SEH sah

Do you have …
¿Padece de …
pah theh seh theh

> palpitations?
> palpitaciones?
> pahl pee tah SYOH nehs

> frequent colds?
> catarros frecuentes?
> kah TAH rrohs freh KWEHN tehs

a constant cough?

tos constante?

tohs kohn STAHN teh

Can you describe what you cough up?

¿Puede describirme lo que suelta?

PWEH theh thehs kree VEER meh loh keh
SWEHL tah

What activity causes you to cough?

¿Qué actividad le provoca la tos?

keh_ahk tee vee THAHTH leh proh VOH kah lah
tohs

What time of day do you cough most?

¿En qué parte del día tiene más accesos de tos?

ehn keh PAHR teh thehl THEE ah TYEH neh
mahs ahk SEH sohs theh tohs

Do you have pain when you cough?

¿La tos le provoca dolor?

lah tohs leh proh VOH kah doh LOHR

Do you breathe easier after coughing?

¿Respira mejor después de toser?

rrehs PEE rah meh HOHR thehs PWEHS theh
toh SEHR

Does sitting or lying down make it better or worse?

¿Crece o mengua el dolor cuando se sienta o se
acuesta?

KREH seh_oh MEHN gwah_ehl doh LOHR
KWAHN doh seh SYEHN tah_oh seh_ah KWEHS
tah

Have you ever had …
¿Alguna vez …
ahl GOO nah vehs

> swelling in your …
> se le han hinchado …
> seh leh ahn een CHAH thoh
>
> bluish color in your …
> se le han puesto morados …
> seh leh ahn PWEHS toh moh RAH thohs
>
> coldness in your …
> se le han quedado fríos …
> seh leh ahn keh THAH thoh FREE ohs
>
>> feet?
>> los pies?
>> lohs pyehs
>>
>> lips?
>> los labios?
>> lohs LAH vyohs
>>
>> hands?
>> las manos?
>> lahs MAH nohs

If your question is about the hands, "blue" and "cold" will be *moradas* and *frías*.

Eye, Ear, Nose, and Throat (EENT)

The questions that follow will give you an overview of EENT problems the patient may have.

Do you have now or have you ever had …
¿Tiene ahora o ha tenido alguna vez …
TYEH neh_ah OH rah_oh_ah teh NEE thoh_ahl
GOO nah vehs

frequent or severe …
frecuente o severamente …
freh KWEHN teh_oh seh veh rah MEHN teh

headaches?
dolor de cabeza?
doh LOHR theh kah VEH sah

earaches?
dolor del oído?
doh LOHR theh_oh EE thoh

colds?
catarros?
kah TAH rrohs

burning of your eyes?
ardor en los ojos?
ahr THOHR ehn lohs OH hohs

crust formation in your eyes?
depósitos en el rabillo del ojo?
deh POH see tohs ehn ehl rrah
VEE yoh thehl OH hoh

itching of your eyes?
picazón en los ojos?
ee kah SOHN ehn lohs OH hohs

tearing of your eyes?
lagrimeo de los ojos?
lah gree MEH oh theh lohs OH
hohs

redness of your eyes?
enrojecimiento de los ojos?
ehn roh heh see MYEHN toh
theh lohs OH hohs

many nosebleeds?
sangrado por la nariz?
sahn GRAH thoh pohr lah
nah REES

many ear infections?
infecciones del oído?
een fehk SYOH nehs thehl oh
EE thoh

trouble breathing through
your nose?
dificultad al respirar por la
nariz?
thee fee kool TAHTH ahl
rrehs pee RAHR pohr lah nah
REES

pain ...
dolor ...
doh LOHR

in your forehead?
en la frente?
ehn lah FREHN teh

under your eyes?
debajo de los ojos?
theh VAH hoh theh lohs OH
hohs

gums that bleed easily?
encías que sangran fácil-
mente?
ehn SEE ahs keh SAHN
grahn FAH seel MEHN teh

recurring sores ...
úlceras frecuentes ...
OOL seh rahs freh KWEHN tehs

on your tongue?
en la lengua?
ehn lah LEHN gwah

in your mouth?
en la boca?
ehn lah VOH kah

Do you have pain when you bend your neck?
¿Le da dolor al flexionar el cuello?
leh thah doh LOHR ahl flehk syoh NAHR ehl
KWEH yoh

Do you have any loss of hearing?
¿Ha notado que oye menos que antes?
ah noh TAH thoh keh_OH yeh MEH nohs
keh_AHN tehs

I am going to clean your ears out with a water flush.
Voy a limpiarle los oídos con agua y esta perilla.
boy ah leem PYAHR leh lohs oh EE thohs kohn
AH gwah_ee_EHS tah peh REE yah

Can you hear this?
¿Puede oír esto?
PWEH theh_oh EER EHS toh

Is it equal in both ears?
¿Se oye igual en los dos oídos?
seh_OH yeh_ee GWAHL ehn lohs thohs oh EE thohs

When was the last time you had a ...
¿Cuándo fue su último examen de ...
KWAHN doh fweh soo_OOL tee moh_ehk SAH mehn deh

> vision test?
> la vista?
> lah VEES tah
>
> hearing test?
> los oídos?
> lohs oh EE thohs

Endocrine System

Have you had ...
¿Ha notado usted ...
ah noh TAH thoh_oos TEHTH

> any problem concentrating?
> problemas con la concentración?
> proh VLEH mahs kohn lah kohn sehn trah SYOHN
>
> any problem sleeping?
> problemas con el sueño?
> proh VLEH mahs kohn ehl SWEH nyoh
>
> any increase in the size of your breasts?
> que se le han aumentado los senos?
> keh seh leh ahn ow mehn TAH thoh lohs SEH nohs

secretions from your nipples?
secreciones de los pezones?
seh creh SYOH nehs theh lohs peh SOH nehs

a change in …
un cambio de …
oon KAHM byoh theh

> your facial features?
> sus rasgos faciales?
> soos RRAHS gohs fah SYAH lehs
>
> your facial hair growth?
> el crecimiento de pelo en su cara?
> ehl kreh see MYEHN toh theh PEH loh_ehn soo KAH rah
>
> the quantity of your body hair?
> la cantidad de pelo por todo el cuerpo?
> lah kahn tee THAHTH deh PEH loh pohr TOH thoh_ehl KWEHR poh
>
> the quantity of the hair on your head?
> la cantidad de su cabello?
> lah kahn tee THAHTH deh soo kah VEH yoh
>
> the color of your hair?
> el color de su pelo?
> ehl koh LOHR theh soo PEH loh

the texture of your hair?
la consistencia de su pelo?
lah kohn sees TEHN syah theh
soo PEH loh

the distribution of your hair?
la distribución de su pelo?
lah dees tree voo SYOHN theh
soo PEH loh

your periods?
la regla menstrual?
lah RREH glah mehns
TRWAHL

your skin tone or texture?
el tono o la consistencia de la
piel?
ehl TOH noh_oh lah kohn sees
TEHN syah theh lah pyehl

the tone of your voice (higher
or lower)?
un tono más alto o bajo de su
voz?
oon TOH noh mahs AHL
toh_oh VAH hoh theh soo vohs

your sensitivity to cold (heat)?
su sensibilidad al frío (calor)?
soo sehn see vee lee THAHTH
ahl FREE_oh (kah LOHR)

Have you noticed that you ...
¿Se ha dado cuenta de que ...
seh ah THAH thoh KWEHN tah theh keh

> are more tired?
> se cansa más?
> seh KAHN sah mahs

> are more nervous?
> se pone más nervioso?
> seh POH neh mahs nehr VYOH soh

> are more thirsty?
> tiene más sed?
> TYEH neh mahs sehth

> perspire more than usual ...
> suda más de lo normal ...
> SOO thah mahs theh loh nohr MAHL

>> during the day?
>> durante el día?
>> doo RAHN teh_ehl
>> THEE ah

>> at night?
>> durante la noche?
>> doo RAHN teh lah NOH
>> cheh

> urinate more?
> orina más?
> oh REE nah mahs

> eat more?
> come más?
> KOH meh mahs

eat more and do not gain weight?
come más sin subir de peso?
KOH meh mahs seen soo BEER theh PEH soh

are confused?
se confunde?
seh kohn FOON deh

Does anyone in your family have diabetes?
¿Tiene diabetes algún familiar suyo?
TYEH neh dyah VEH tehs ahl GOON fah mee
LYAHR SOO yoh

Gastrointestinal System

How many servings of each of these do you have
each week?
¿Cuántas raciones de estos toma usted cada semana?
KWAHN tahs rrah SYOH nehs theh_EHS tohs
TOH mah_oos TEHTH KAH thah seh MAH nah

alcohol	bebidas alcohólicas	beh VEE thahs ahl koh OH lee kahs
coffee	café	kah FEH
milk	leche	LEH cheh
soft drinks	refrescos	rreh FREHS kohs
water	agua	AH gwah

Do you get indigestion from any foods? Which ones?
¿Le provoca una indigestión alguna comida? ¿Cuál?
leh proh VOH kah_OO nah_een dee hehs
TYOHN ahl GOO nah koh MEE thah kwahl

Is there any food you cannot eat?
¿Hay alguna comida que no puede comer?
ay ahl GOO nah koh MEE thah keh noh PWEH theh koh MEHR

Do you have a good appetite?
¿Tiene buen apetito?
TYEH neh bwehn ah peh TEE toh

Has your weight …
¿Su peso ha …
soo PEH soh_ah

> increased?
> subido?
> soo VEE thoh

> decreased?
> bajado?
> vah HAH thoh

>> How much?
>> ¿Cuánto?
>> KWAHN toh

Are you on a special diet?
¿Está a una dieta especial?
ehs TAH_ah_OO nah DYEH tah ehs peh SYAHL

Do you often …
¿Tiene frecuentemente …
TYEH neh freh kwehn teh MEHN teh

> burp?
> eructos?
> eh ROOK tohs

pass gas?
mucho flato? (muchos pedos?)
MOO choh FLAH toh / MOO chohs PEH thohs

feel nauseated?
náuseas?
NOW seh ahs

vomit?
vómitos?
VOH mee tohs

Do you wake up with heartburn?
¿Amanece con el ardor de la indigestión?
ah mah NEH seh kohn ehl ahr THOHR theh
lah_een dee hehs TYOHN

How often?
¿Con qué frecuencia?
kohn keh freh KWEHN syah

Have you noticed ...
¿Se ha notado ...
seh ah noh TAH thoh

   a change in the color of your urine?
   un cambio del color de la orina?
   oon KAHM byoh thehl koh LOHR theh lah_oh
   REE nah

   blood on the toilet paper?
   sangre en el papel higiénico?
   SAHN greh_ehn ehl pah PEHL ee HYEH
   nee koh

   your stools ...
   que su materia fecal ...
   keh soo mah TEH ryah feh KAHL

have mucus?
tiene moco?
TYEH neh MOH koh

are black?
es negra?
ehs NEH grah

are bloody?
tiene sangre?
TYEH neh SAHN greh

are unusual-smelling?
tiene olor fétido?
TYEH neh_oh LOHR FEH tee thoh

are clay-colored?
tiene el color de arcilla?
TYEH neh_ehl koh LOHR theh_ahr SEE yah

Have you had any change in your bowel habits?
¿Ha notado algún cambio en su defecación normal?
ah noh TAH thoh_ahl GOON KAHM byoh_ehn soo deh feh kah SYOHN nohr MAHL

When did it start?
¿Cuándo empezó?
KWAHN doh_ehm peh SOH

Muscular/Skeletal System

Did this happen during ...
¿Esto ocurrió porque ...
EHS toh_oh koo RRYOH POHR keh

exercise?
hacía ejercicio?
ah SEE ah_eh hehr SEE syoh

a fall?
se cayó?
seh kah YOH

normal activity?
hacía actividades normales?
ah SEE ah_ahk tee vee THAH thehs nohr
MAH lehs

Has this happened before?
¿Esto le ha ocurrido antes?
EHS toh leh_ah_oh koo RREE thoh_AHN tehs

Use the following commands to elicit specific
movements. Note that some movement commands
change according to what's being moved. In general, attaching *SE* to the end of a command shifts
the action to the whole person rather than a limb.
Compare: *Levante el brazo*, Raise your arm; *Levántese*,
Raise yourself (freely, get up, sit up, stand up).

Raise your ...	Levante su ...	leh VAHN teh soo
Lower your ...	Baje su ...	BAH heh soo
Push.	Empuje.	ehm POO heh
Pull.	Tire.	TEE reh
Rotate your ... (limb)	Gire su ...	HEE reh soo
Rotate. (self)	Gírese.	HEE reh seh
Bend. (all-purpose)	Doble.	DOH vleh

continues

continued

| Straighten your ... (limb) | Enderezca su | ehn deh REH seh |
| Straighten. (self) | Yérgase. | YEHR gah seh |

Neurological System

Do you have ...
¿Tiene ...
TYEH neh

blind spots?
manchas negras delante de los ojos?
MAHN chahs NEH grahs theh LAHN teh
theh lohs OH hohs

blurred vision?
la vista borrosa?
lah VEES tah voh RROH sah

double vision?
visión doble?
vee SYOHN DOH vleh

spots before your eyes?
manchas delante de los ojos?
MAHN chahs theh LAHN teh theh lohs OH
hohs

pain behind your eyes?
dolor en los ojos?
doh LOHR ehn lohs OH hohs

tingling?
un hormigueo?
oon ohr mee GEH oh

numbness?
entumecimiento?
ehn too meh see MYEHN toh

paralysis?
parálisis?
pah RAH lee sees

Do you have a loss …
¿Experimenta una pérdida …
ehs peh ree MEHN tah_OO nah PEHR thee thah

of feeling in your face?
de sensación en la cara?
theh sehn sah SYOHN ehn lah KAH rah

of taste?
del gusto para la comida?
thehl GOOS toh PAH rah lah koh MEE thah

feeling heat (cold) on your skin?
sentir el calor o el frío por la piel?
sehn TEER ehl kah LOHR oh_ehl FREE oh
pohr lah pyehl

Do you have …
¿Experimenta …
ehks peh ree MEHN tah

a sensation of odd or unpleasant odors?
una sensación de olores malos o desagradables?
OO nah sehn sah SYOHN theh_oh LOH rehs
MAH lohs oh deh sah grah THAH vlehs

a sensation of odd or unpleasant tastes?
una sensación de sabores malos o desagradables?
OO nah sehn sah SYOHN theh sah VOH rehs
MAH lohs oh deh sah grah THAH vlehs

trouble swallowing?
dificultad para tragar?
thee fee kool TAHTH PAH rah trah GAHR

dizziness?
mareo?
mah REH oh

Convulsions and Headaches

Do you have convulsions?
¿Padece de convulsiones?
pah THEH seh theh kohm bool SYOH nehs

When did you have your first (last) convulsion?
¿Cuándo tuvo su primera (última) convulsión?
KWAHN doh TOO voh soo pree MEH rah (OOL
tee mah) kohm bool SYOHN

How often do you have them?
¿Con qué frecuencia le vienen?
kohn keh freh KWEHN syah leh VYEH nehn

Are they preceded by …
¿Están precedidas por …
ehs THAN preh seh THEE thahs pohr

a special odor?
un olor especial?
oon oh LOHR ehs peh SYAHL

a vision?
una visión?
OO nah vee SYOHN

When you convulse, do you ...
Al sufrir una convulsión, ...
ahl soo FREER OO nah kohm bool SYOHN

> lose consciousness?
> ¿pierde el conocimiento?
> PYEHR theh_ehl koh noh see MYEHN toh

How long does each convulsion last?
¿Cuánto dura cada convulsión?
KWAHN toh THOO rah KAH thah kohm bool
SYOHN

After a convulsion, how long are you usually ...
Pasada la convulsión, ¿por cuánto tiempo queda ...
pah SAH thah lah kohm bool SYOHN, pohr
KWAHN toh TYEHM poh KEH thah

> unconscious?
> inconsciente?
> een kohn SYEHN teh

> disoriented?
> desorientado?
> deh soh ryehn TAH thoh

Does anything bring it on?
¿Hay algo que provoque la convulsión?
ay AHL goh keh proh VOH keh lah kohm bool
SYOHN

Pediatrics

We will record the baby's weight (height) in ...
Apuntaremos el peso (tamaño) del bebé en ...
ah poon tah REH mohs ehl PEH soh (tah
MAH nyoh) thehl veh VEH_ehn

grams	gramos	GRAH mohs
ounces	onzas	OHN sahs
pounds	libras	LEE vrahs
inches	pulgadas	pool GAH thahs
centimeters	centímetros	sehn TEE meh trohs

Does (s)he have pain?
¿Tiene dolor?
TYEH neh doh LOHR

How did the injury happen?
¿Cómo se lastimó?
KOH moh seh lahs tee MOH

Is he (she) sick?
¿Está enfermo (enferma)?
ehs TAH_ehn FEHR moh

Does (s)he ...

burp?	¿Eructa?	eh ROOK tah
cough?	¿Tose?	TOH seh
crawl?	¿Gatea?	gah TEH ah
cry often?	¿Llora a menudo?	YOH rah_ah meh NOO thoh
drink milk?	¿Toma leche?	TOH mah LEH cheh

eat well?	¿Come bien?	KOH meh vyehn
talk?	¿Habla?	AH vlah
walk?	¿Camina?	kah MEE nah

Does (s)he cry for no apparent reason?
¿Llora sin razón aparente?
YOH rah seen rrah SOHN ah pah REHN teh

Is he (she) constipated?
¿Está estreñido (estreñida)?
ehs TAH_ehs treh NYEE thoh

Does (s)he have diarrhea?
¿Tiene diarrea?
TYEH neh dyah RREH ah

How often does the baby spit up?
¿Con qué frecuencia regurgita el bebé?
kohn keh freh KWEHN syah reh goor HEE tah_
ehl veh VEH

Does s(he) have vomiting?
¿Vomita?
boh MEE tah

Are there any feeding problems?
¿Hay algún problema con su alimentación?
ay ahl GOON proh VLEH mah kohn soo_ah lee
mehn tah SYOHN

Sexually Transmitted Diseases

Do you get recurring sores on your genitals?
¿Le salen heridas recurrentes en el sexo?
leh SAH lehn eh REE thahs rreh koo RREHN teh
ehn ehl SEHK soh

Where?
¿Dónde?
DOHN deh

> With an infection on your genitals, do you
> have ...
> ¿La infección en sus genitales le provoca ...
> lah_een fehk SYOHN ehn soos heh nee TAH
> lehs leh proh VOH kah

any discharge?	cualquier descarga	kwahl KYEHR thehs KAHR gah
burning?	ardor?	ahr THOHR
itching?	picazón?	pee kah SOHN
redness?	enrojecimiento?	ehn roh heh see MYEHN toh
sores?	heridas?	eh REE thahs
swelling?	hinchazón?	een chah SOHN
tenderness?	sensibilidad?	sehn sah vee lee THAHTH

Urinary Tract

Do you have pain ...
¿Tiene dolor ...
TYEH neh doh LOHR

> in your upper back?
> de riñones?
> theh rree NYOH nehs
> on urination?
> al orinar?
> ahl oh ree NAHR

the whole time?
durante toda la descarga?
doo RAHN teh TOH thah lah thehs KAHR gah

How soon after intercourse does the burning, pain,
or urgency start?
Después del roce sexual, ¿cuánto tarda en comenzar el ardor, el dolor, o la urgencia?
dehs PWEHS thehl RROH seh sehk SWAHL,
KWAHN toh TAHR thah_ehn koh mehn SAHR
ehl ahr THOHR, ehl doh LOHR, oh lah_oor
HEHN syah

Do you urinate in larger or smaller quantities than
you used to?
¿El volumen de su orina es mayor o menor que
antes orinaba?
ehl voh LOO mehn deh soo_oh REE nah_ehs mah
YOHR oh meh NOHR keh_AHN tehs oh ree
NAH vah

Do you urinate a lot at night?
¿Orina mucho en la noche?
oh REE nah MOO choh_ehn lah NOH cheh

Do you often have …
¿Tiene a menudo …
TYEH neh_ah meh NOO thoh

an urgency to urinate?
una urgencia de orinar?
OO nah_oor HEHN syah theh_oh ree NAHR

difficulty starting the urinary stream?
dificultad para iniciar el chorro?
thee fee kool TAHTH PAH rah_ee nee
SYAHR ehl CHOH rroh

an interrupted stream?

el chorro interrumpido?

ehl CHOH rroh_een teh rroom PEE thoh

dribbling after urination?

goteo al terminar de orinar?

goh TEH oh_ahl tehr mee NAHR theh_oh
ree NAHR

small stones in your urine?

arenilla en la orina?

ah reh NEE yah_ehn lah_oh REE nah

cloudy urine?

la orina turbia?

lah_oh REE nah TOOR vyah

pink urine?

la orina rosada?

lah_oh REE nah rroh SAH thah

Chapter 6

Diagnostic Tests and Procedures

Few patients actually look forward to diagnostic tests and procedures. The equipment may be unfamiliar and intimidating, and the process can be confusing or downright painful. Add to that a language barrier, and you've got a recipe for fear.

In this chapter, you'll find words and phrases to help you explain tests, procedures, and preps to your Spanish-speaking patients, and to reassure and guide them as the procedure is performed. For the patient, understanding what it's all about makes it far easier to submit to whatever must be done.

What the Doctor Ordered

Before examining the comprehensive list of specific diagnostic tests, for quick reference, take a look at the umbrella words for basic types of tests. Because of the similarities between Spanish and English medical terms, you will easily recognize the medical terms attached to these important roots.

Just What the Doctor Ordered

function test	una prueba funcional de	OO nah PRWEH vah foon syoh NAHL theh
analysis	un análisis	oon ah NAH lee sees
biopsy	una biopsia	OO nah BYOHP sya
culture	un cultivo	oon kool TEE voh
examination	un examen	oon ehk SAH mehn
scan	una toma axial computerizada	OO nah TOH mah_ahk SYAHL kohm poo teh ree SAH thah
surgery	una cirugía	OO nah see roo HEE ah
test	una prueba	OO nah PRWEH vah
x-ray	una radiografía	OO nah rrah thyoh grah FEE ah

Here are the names of many common medical tests and procedures. To help you discuss them with your patients, less technical descriptions are included where the Spanish translations of the names don't fully explain the tests:

adrenal function test
una prueba de función adrenal
OO nah PRWEH vah theh foon SYOHN ah threh NAHL

angiogram
un angiograma
oon ahn hyoh GRAH mah

(visualization of an organ through veins and arteries)
(visualización de un órgano a través de venas y
arterias)
(vee swah lee sah SYOHN theh_oon OHR gah noh_ah
trah VEHS theh VEH nahs ee ahr TEH ryahs)

arteriogram
un arteriograma
oon ahr teh ryoh GRAH mah
(x-ray of the arteries)
(una radiografía de las arterias)
(OO nah rrah thyoh grah FEE ah theh lahs ahr TEH
ryahs)

barium enema
una enema de bario
OO nah_eh NEH mah theh BAh ryoh
(lower bowel X-ray)
(una radiografía del intestino grueso)
(OO nah rah thyoh gra FEE ah thehl een tehs TEE
noh GRWEH soh)

barium swallow
un trago de bario
oon TRAH goh theh BAH ryoh
(upper digestive tract X-ray)
(una radiografía del esófago y estómago)
(OO nah rrah thyoh grah FEE ah thehl eh SOH fah
Goh ee ehs TOH mah goh)

biopsy
una biopsia
OO na BYOP syah
(tissue sample test)
(examen de una porción de tejido humano)
(ehk SAH mehn theh OO na pohr SYOHN theh teh
HEE thoh_hoo MAH noh)

bladder catheterization
cateterismo de la vejiga
kah teh teh REES moh theh lah veh HEE gah
(soft tube in the bladder)
(introducción de un tubito blando en la vejiga)
(een troh dook SYOHN theh oon too BEE to
BLAHN doh_ehn lah veh HEE gah)

blood test
un análisis de la sangre
oon ah NAH lee sees theh lah SAHN greh

bronchoscopy
una broncoscopía
OO nah brohn kohs koh PEE ah
(scope exam of the bronchial tubes)
(examen visual de los bronquios)
(ehk SAH mehn bee SWAHL theh lohs BROHN
kyohs)

renal function test
una prueba de la función de los riñones
OO nah PRWEH vah theh lah foon SYOHN theh
lohs rree NYOH nehs

cardiac catheterization
un cateterismo cardíaco
oon kah teh teh REES moh kahr DEE ah koh
(invasive procedure to open clogged arteries)
(procedimiento invasivo para ensanchar arterias
bloqueadas)
(proh seh thee MYEHN toh_eem bah SEE voh
PAH rah_ehn sahn chahr ahr TEH ryahs bloh keh
AH thahs)

cardiac enzymes test
una prueba de enzimas cardíacas
OO nah PRWEH vah theh_ehn SEE mahs kahr
THEE ah kahs
(heart attack confirmation)
(para confirmar un ataque del corazón)
(PAH rah kohn feer MAHR oon ah TAH keh thehl
koh rah SOHN)

cardioversion
una cardioversión
OO na kahr thyoh vehr SYOHN
(restoration to normal heart rhythm)
(restablecimiento del ritmo normal del corazón)
(rrehs tah vleh see MYEHN toh thehl RREET
moh nohr MAHL thehl koh rah SOHN)

CAT/CT scan
una tomografía computerizada
OO nah toh moh grah FEE ah kohm poo teh ree
SAH thah
(painless view inside the body, like an X-ray)
(toma sin dolor de una vista interior del cuerpo,
como una radiografía)
(TOH mah seen doh LOHR theh_OO nah VEES
tah_een teh RYOHR thehl KWEHR poh, KOH
moh_OO nah rrah thyoh grah FEE ah)

cholecystogram
un colecistograma
oon koh leh sees toh GRAH mah
(gall bladder x-ray)
(radiografía de la vesícula biliar)
(rrah thyoh grah FEE ah theh lah veh SEE koo lah
vee LYAHR)

colonoscopy
una colonoscopía
OO na koh loh nohs koh PEE ah
(scope exam of the lower tract)
(examen visual del colon mediante un tubo)
(ehk SAH mehn bee SWAHL thehl KOH lohn
meh DYAHN teh_oon TOO voh)

CBC (complete blood count)
un análisis completo de la sangre
oon ah NAH lee sees kohm PLEH toh theh lah
SAHN greh

culture
un cultivo
oon kool TEE voh

cystoscopy
una cistoscopía
OO nah sees tohs koh PEE ah
(scope exam of the bladder)
(examen visual de la vejiga mediante un tubo)
(ehk SAH mehn vee SWAHL theh lah veh HEE
gah meh DYAHN teh_oon TOO voh)

echocardiogram
un ecocardiograma
oon eh koh kahr thyoh GRAH mah
(ultrasound exam of the heart)
(examen ultrasónico del corazón)
(ehk SAH mehn ool trah SOH nee koh thehl koh
rah SOHN)

EEG/electroencephalogram
electroencefalograma
eh lehk troh ehn seh fah loh GRAH mah

(record of brain's electrical activity)
(gráfico de la actividad eléctrica del cerebro)
(GRAH fee koh theh lah_ahk tee vee THAHTH
eh LEHK tree kah thehl seh REH broh)

ECG/electrocardiogram
un electrocardiograma
oon eh lehk tro kahr thyoh GRAH mah
(record of heart's electrical activity)
(gráfico de la actividad eléctrica del corazón)
(GRAH fee koh theh lah_ahk tee vee THAHTH
eh LEHK tree kah thehl koh rah SOHN)

endoscopy
una endoscopía
OO nah_ehn dohs koh PEE ah
(scope exam of the stomach)
(examen visual del estómago mediante un tubo)
(ehk SAH mehn bee SWAHL thehl ehs TOH mah
goh meh THYAHN teh_oon TOO voh)

exercise/stress tolerance test
una prueba de tolerancia al ejercicio físico
OO nah PRWEH vah theh toh leh RAHN
syah_ahl eh hehr SEE syoh FEE see koh

eye test
examen de la vista
ehk SAH mehn theh lah VEES tah

glucose tolerance test
(special blood sugar test that takes four hours)
una prueba de tolerancia a la glucosa que requiere
cuatro horas
OO nah PRWEH vah theh toh leh RAHN syah_ah
lah gloo KOH sah keh rreh KYEH reh KWAH
troh_OH rahs

hearing test
examen de la audición
ehk SAH mehn deh_ow thee SYOHN

kidney biopsy
una biopsia del riñón
OO nah BYOHP syah thehl ree NYOHN

liver function test
una prueba funcional del hígado
OO nah PRWEH vah foon syoh NAHL thehl EE
gah thoh

mammogram
mamograma
mah moh GRAH mah
(x-ray exam of the breasts)
(radiografía de los senos)
(rrah thyoh grah FEE ah theh lohs SEH nohs)

MRI/magnetic resonance imaging
Imagen por resonancia magnética
ee MAH hehn pohr rreh soh NAHN syah mahg
NEH tee kah
(painless view inside the body)
(para visualizar sin dolor el interior del cuerpo)
(PAH rah vee swah lee SAHR seen doh LOHR ehl
een teh RYOHR thehl KWEHR poh)

ovarian function test
una prueba funcional de los ovarios
OO nah PRWEH vah foon syoh NAHL theh lohs
oh VAH ryohs

pancreatic function test
una prueba funcional del páncreas
OO nah PRWEH vah foon syoh NAHL thehl
PAHN kreh ahs

parathyroid function test
una prueba funcional paratiroidea
OO nah PRWEH vah foon syoh NAHL PAH rah
tee roy THEH ah

pituitary function test
una prueba funcional pituitaria
OO nah PRWEH vah foon syoh NAHL pee twee
TAH ryah

PPD test (tuberculosis test)
una prueba para tuberculosis
OO nah PRWEH vah PAH rah too vehr koo LOH
sees

proctoscopy
proctoscopía
prohk tohs koh PEE ah
(scope exam of the rectum/anal area)
(examen del área del recto)
(ehk SAH mehn thehl AH ryah thehl REHK toh)

scan
visualización electrónica del interior del cuerpo
bee swah lee sah SYOHN eh lehk TROH nee kah
thel een teh RYOHR thehl KWEHR poh

sigmoidoscopy
sigmoidoscopía
seeg moy thohs koh pee ah
(partial scope exam of the lower tract)
(examen visual del colon)
(ehk SAH mehn bee SWAHL thehl KOH lohn)

sonogram
sonograma
soh noh GRAH mah
(painless view inside the body)
(visualización sin dolor del interior del cuerpo)
(bee swah lee sah SYOHN seen doh LOHR thehl
een teh RYOHR thehl KWEHR poh)

sputum test
examen del esputo/de la flema
ehk SAH mehn thehl ehs POO toh/theh lah FLEH
mah

stool test
examen del excremento
ehk SAH mehn thehl ehs kreh MEHN toh

surgery
cirugía
see roo HEE ah

thyroid function test
una prueba funcional de la tiroides
OO nah PRWEH vah foon syoh NAHL theh lah
tee ROY thehs

ultrasound
ultrasonido
ool trah soh NEE thoh
(painless view inside the body using sound waves)
(un examen ultrasónico sin dolor del interior del
cuerpo)
(oon ehk SAH mehn ool trah SOH nee koh seen
doh LOHR thehl een teh RYOHR thehl KWEHR
poh)

upper GI series
una serie gastrointestinal superior
OO nah SEH ryeh gahs troh een tehs tee NAHL soo
peh RYOHR
(x-rays of the upper digestive tract)
(radiografías de la parte superior del tracto alimenticio)
(rrah thyoh grah FEE ahs theh lah PAHR teh soo peh
RYOHR thehl TRAHK toh_ah lee mehn TEE syoh)

urine test
un análisis de la orina
oon ah NAH lee sees theh lah_oh REE nah

x-ray
radiografía
rrah thyoh grah FEE ah

Guiding the Patient Through It

These phrases are useful before, during, and after
many tests and procedures, for doctors and techni-
cians alike:

You need to have_____.
Necesita_____.
neh seh SEE tah

You are going to have _____.
Le van a hacer_____.
leh vahn ah_ah SEHR

We need more information.
Necesitamos más información.
neh seh SEE tah mohs mahs een fohr mah SYOHN

This test will provide that information.
Esta prueba nos dará esa información.
EHS tah PRWEH vah nohs dah RAH_EH
sah_een fohr mah SYOHN

Your doctor has ordered this test for you.
Su doctor le ha mandado hacer esta prueba.
soo dohk TOHR leh_ah mahn DAH thoh_ah
SEHR EHS tah PRWEH vah

This will give us more information about
your_____.
Esto nos dará más información sobre su_____.
EHS toh nohs dará thah RAH mahs een fohr mah
SYOHN soh vreh soo

Please follow these instructions before you come
for the test.
Antes de hacerse la prueba, siga usted estas instruc-
ciones al pie de la letra.
AHN tehs theh_ah SEHR seh lah PRWEH vah,
SEE gah_oos TEHTH EHS tahs eens trook
SYOH nehs ahl pyeh theh lah LEH trah

You must fast for _____ hours before this test.
Tiene que ayunar por _____ horas antes de esta
prueba.
TYEH neh keh_ah yoo NAHR pohr _____ OH
rahs AHN tehs theh_EHS tah PRWEH vah

Don't eat or drink anything after midnight.
No coma ni tome nada después de la medianoche.
noh KOH mah nee TOH meh NAH thah thehs
PWEHS theh lah meh dyah NOH cheh

Put your _____ here.
Ponga _____ aquí.
POHN gah_____ ah KEE

Please don't move until I tell you to.
No se mueva hasta que le diga.
noh seh MWEH vah_AHS tah keh leh THEE gah

Please lie down on the table.
Échese en la mesa.
EH cheh seh_ehn lah MEH sah

Are you comfortable?
¿Está usted cómodo?
ehs TAH_oos TEHTH KOH moh doh

Are you warm enough?
¿Tiene frío?
TYEH neh FREE oh

I need to prep this area.
Necesito preparar esta área.
neh seh SEE toh preh pah RAHR EHS tah_AH
reh ah

I'm going to start an IV for medication.
Voy a ponerle una infusión intravenosa para sus
medicinas.
boy ah poh NEHR leh_OO nah_een foo SYOHN
een trah veh NOH sah PAH rah soos meh thee
SEE nahs

Breathe slowly.
Respire despacio.
rrehs PEE reh thehs PAH syoh

Breathe normally.
Respire normalmente.
rrehs PEE reh nohr mahl MEHN teh

Take a deep breath and hold it.
Aspire profundamente y aguante el aliento.
ahs PEE reh proh foon dah MEHN teh ee ah
GWAHN teh_ehl ah LYEHN toh

You can breathe now.
Puede respirar ahora.
PWEH theh rrehs pee RAHR ah OH rah

You can relax now.
Puede relajarse ahora.
PWEH theh rreh lah HAHR seh_ah OH rah

That's all—we're done.
¡Eso es todo! Hemos terminado.
EH soh_ehs TOH thoh EH mohs tehr mee NAH
thoh

Keep the bandage on for ____.
Debe llevar la venda por ____.
DEH veh yeh VAHR lah VEHN dah pohr

Don't try to drive today.
No trate de manejar el automóvil hoy.
noh TRAH teh theh mah neh HAHR ehl ow toh
MOH veel oy

Call the doctor if anything happens.
Llame al doctor si pasa cualquier cosa.
YAH meh_ahl dohk TOHR see PAH sah kwahl
kyehr KOH sah

It will take a few days to get the results.
Tardarán unos días en mandarnos los resultados.
tahr thah RAHN OO nohs THEE ahs ehn mahn
DAHR nohs lohs rreh sool TAH thohs

We will call you with the results.
Le avisaremos por teléfono cuando tengamos los
resultados.
leh_ah vee sah REH mohs pohr teh LEH foh noh
KWAHN doh tehn GAH mohs lohs rreh sool TAH
thohs

We will mail you the results.
Le enviaremos los resultados por correo.
leh_ehm byah REH mohs lohs rreh sool TAH thohs
pohr koh RREH oh

Call this number for the results.
Llame a este número para obtener los resultados.
YAH meh_ah_EHS teh NOO meh roh PAH rah
ohv teh NEHR lohs rreh sool TAH thohs

I will send the information to your doctor.
Voy a mandarle la información a su doctor.
boy ah mahn DAHR leh lah_een fohr mah SYOHN
ah soo dohk TOHR

For the Lab

I need to take blood from your arm.
Necesito sacarle sangre de su brazo.
neh seh SEE toh sah KAHR leh SAHN greh theh
soo BRAH soh

Please make a fist.
Haga un puño, por favor.
AH gah_oon POO nyoh, pohr fah VOHR

You can open your hand now.
Ahora puede abrir la mano.
ah OH rah PWEH theh_ah VREER lah MAH noh

Hold your arm up.
Mantenga el brazo elevado.
mahn TEHN gah_ehl BRAH soh_eh leh VAH thoh

Press on this.
Presione esto.
preh SYOH neh_EHS toh

I need to take a swab from here.
Necesito tomarle una muestra de aquí con esto.
neh seh SEE toh toh MAHR leh_OO nah
MWEHS trah theh_ah KEE kohn EHS toh

Cough some sputum into this.
Tosa y escupa en esto lo que salga.
TOH sah ee ehs KOO pah_ehn EHS toh loh keh
SAHL gah

We need a urine specimen.
Necesitamos un espécimen de su orina.
neh seh see TAH mohs oon ehs PEH see mehn
theh soo_oh REE nah

For Cardiovascular Tests

I need to put this (these) on you.
Tengo que ponerle esto(s).
TEHN goh keh poh NEHR leh_EHS toh(s)

It will start slowly.
Se pone en marcha lentamente.
seh POH neh_ehn MAHR chah lehn tah MEHN teh

It will get faster now.
Ahora acelera.
ah OH rah_ah seh LEH rah

Tell me when you are too tired to continue.
Avíseme cuando se canse tanto que no puede continuar.
ah VEE seh meh KWAHN doh seh KAHN seh
TAHN toh keh noh PWEH theh kohn tee NWAHR

You need to wear this for 24 hours.
Tendrá que llevar esto por veinticuatro horas.
tehn DRAH keh yeh VAHR EHS toh pohr veyn tee
KWAH troh_OH rahs

Go about your usual activities.
No cambie sus actividades. Siga haciéndolo todo
como de costumbre.
noh KAHM bych soos ahk tee vee THAH thehs.
SEE gah_ah SYEHN doh loh TOH thoh KOH moh
theh kohs TOOM breh

Do not get this wet.
No permita que esto se moje.
noh pehr MEE tah keh EHS toh seh MOH heh

For Biopsies

We need a biopsy (a small sample of tissue) of _____.
Necesitamos una biopsia (una pequeña muestra de
tejido) de _____.
neh seh see TAH mohs OO nah BYOHP syah (OO
nah peh KEH nyah MWEHS trah theh teh HEE
thoh) theh

We'll inject local anesthesia so you feel no pain.
Le vamos a poner una inyección de anestesia local
para que no sienta dolor.

leh VAH mohs ah poh NEHR OO nah_een yehk
SYOHN deh_ah nehs TEH syah loh KAHL PAH rah
keh noh SYEHN tah thoh LOHR

I have to clean the area first.
Tengo que limpiar el área primero.
TEHN goh keh leem PYAHR ehl AH reh ah pree
MEH roh

You'll need to lie on your side.
Tiene que acostarse sobre un costado.
TYEH neh keh_ah kohs TAHR seh SOH vreh oon
kohs TAH thoh

I am sending the sample to the laboratory.
Mando la muestra al laboratorio.
MAHN doh lah MWEHS trah_ahl lah voh rah TOH
ryoh

For Gastrointestinal Tests

Did you empty your bowels for this test?
¿Se evacuó el vientre completamente para este examen?
seh_eh vah KWOH ehl VYEHN treh kohm pleh tah
MEHN teh PAH rah_EHS teh_ehk SAH mehn

Please drink this.
Tómese esto, por favor.
TOH meh seh_EHS toh, pohr fah VOHR

I'm going to put barium in your lower bowel.
Voy a ponerle bario en el recto.
boy ah poh NEHR leh VAH ryoh_ehn ehl RREHK toh

Hold it as long as you can.
Reténgalo lo más posible.
rreh TEHN gah loh loh mahs poh SEE vleh

The Diagnosis

When giving a diagnosis to an English-speaking patient, professional reserve can be helpful. It's often easier for all to focus on facts, not feelings.

But for Spanish-speaking patients, the same is not true. Unless the diagnosis is strictly routine, your Hispanic patient will look to you for empathy and compassion. In moments of joy or despair, relief or apprehension, Spanish speakers are closest to those they love and trust. You are delivering the news, so you are the one they need to trust. To gain that trust, be sure your demeanor allows them that closeness.

Use the phrases in this chapter to convey feelings as well as information, but don't forget body language. Especially in the case of bad news, that can mean standing very close, gently cradling the patient's hand, forearm, or elbow, or lightly resting your palm on the patient's shoulder. Direct eye contact is also crucial. Looking elsewhere—even at test results!—suggests to the patient you are being evasive.

Delivering the News

Before you deliver the actual diagnosis, lead in with a phrase that shows understanding and empathy.

First, Show That You Care

Good news!
¡Le tengo buenas noticias!
leh TEHN goh BWEH nahs noh TEE syahs

It's not as good as we had hoped.
No es tan bueno como lo esperábamos.
noh_ehs tahn BWEH noh KOH moh loh_ehs peh RAH vah mohs

I'm (so) sorry to report that ...
Siento (tanto) tener que decirle que ...
SYEHN toh (TAHN toh) teh NEHR keh theh SEER leh keh

The Facts of the Matter

After the patient knows you're speaking from the heart, he or she is better prepared to accept and understand the diagnosis itself. These phrases will help you discuss it:

> This is (insert optional modifier) serious.
> Esto es (...) grave.
> EHS toh ehs (...) GRAH veh

(not very)	poco	POH koh
(somewhat)	algo	AHL goh
(a bit)	un poco	oom POH koh
(rather)	bastante	vahs TAHN teh

This is not (at all) serious.
Esto no es (nada) grave.
EHS toh noh_ehs (NAH thah) GRAH veh

This is (extremely) contagious.
Esto es (extremadamente) contagioso.
EHS toh_ehs (ehs treh mah thah MEHN teh)
kohn tah HYOH soh

This is not contagious.
Esto no es contagioso.
EHS toh noh_ehs kohn tah HYOH soh

We can treat this with medication.
Esto lo podemos tratar con medicamentos.
EHS toh loh poh THEH mohs trah TAHR kohn
meh thee kah MEHN tohs

This will require surgery.
Esto requiere cirujía.
EHS toh rreh KYEH reh see roo HEE ah

(See Chapter 9 for names of common surgical procedures.)

You will need ...
Usted va a necesitar ...
oos TEHTH vah_ah neh seh see TAHR

   a brace.
   una abrazadera.
   OO nah_ah brah sah THEH rah

   a cast.
   un yeso.
   oon YEH soh

physical therapy.
fisioterapia.
fee syoh teh RAH pyah

¡Ojo!

Incurable? If the patient is in deep denial, use the first of the following sentences. If not, the second one stresses the fact that you can help.

We can ease the symptoms, but there is no cure.
Podemos aliviar los síntomas, pero es incurable.
poh THEH mohs ah lee VYAHR lohs SEEN toh mahs, PEH roh ehs een koo RAH vleh

There is no cure, but we can ease the symptoms.
Es incurable, pero podemos aliviar los síntomas.
ehs een koo RAH vleh, PEH roh poh THEH mohs ah lee VYAHR lohs SEEN toh mahs

You need further testing.
Necesita otras pruebas.
neh seh SEE tah_OH trahs PRWEH vahs

You need to see a specialist.
Necesita ver a un especialista.
neh seh SEE tah vehr ah_oon ehs peh syah LEES tah

You don't need to be admitted to the hospital; we can take care of you here.
Usted no necesita internarse; vamos a atenderle aquí.
oos TEHTH noh neh seh SEE tah_een tehr NAHR seh; BAH mohs ah_ah tehn DEHR leh_ah KEE

We can see you as an outpatient.
Podemos atenderle sin hospitalización.
poh THEH mohs ah tehn DEHR leh seen ohs pee tah lee sah SYOHN

Through Their Eyes

Hispanic patients equate hospitalization with the best care possible, so they may think outpatient status means you're (deliberately) offering substandard care. To avoid this impression, use the phrase above rather than saying "We consider you an outpatient."

Follow Up with Feeling

If the news has been bad, some words of encouragement are always welcome, particularly to Spanish speakers. Here are some phrases that will show your heartfelt support. To English speakers some may seem a bit melodramatic, but in Spanish they strike just the right note:

Don't worry.
¡No se preocupe!
noh seh preh_oh KOO peh

Do not be afraid.
¡No tenga miedo!
noh TEHN gah MYEH thoh

Don't give up hope!
¡No se desespere!
noh seh thehs ehs PEH reh

God willing, we'll beat this thing.
Venceremos, si Dios quiere.
behn seh REH mohs see THYOHS KYEH reh

And if the diagnosis is truly bad, don't forget the effect it will have on the patient's family. It will mean much to your patient to ask:

> Will you allow me to help you talk with your family?
> ¿Me permite ayudarle a hablar con su familia?
> meh pehr MEE teh_ah yoo THAHR
> leh_ah_ah VLAHR kohn soo fah MEE lyah

If the patient welcomes this help, and you do speak to the family, be sure to show your concern by using empathetic lead-in phrases with them as well.

Ailments

A book of this size can't possibly list Spanish equivalents for every disease. This section has a representative selection of common ailments. If you need a more exhaustive list, there are excellent medical dictionaries readily available. For cancer-related vocabulary, see the "Cancer" section of this chapter. For more vocabulary on HIV/AIDS, see Chapter 8.

¡Ojo!

The concept of "have" used with various medical conditions may be expressed differently according to the condition.
Three common translations are as follows:

tiene	TYEH neh
padece de	pah THEH seh theh
experimenta	ehs peh ree MEHN tah

Their literal meanings are "you have," "you suffer from," "you are experiencing," respectively.

You have …
Usted tiene …
oos TEHTH TYEH neh

To discuss another person's diagnosis, insert the appropriate relationship word in place of the [blank].

Your [family member] has …
Su […] tiene …
soo […] TYEH neh …

The baby has …
El bebé tiene …
ehl veh VEH TYEH neh …

The problem is …
Se trata de …
seh TRAH tah theh …

Through Their Eyes

To an English speaker, the medical words *demencia* (the illness dementia) and *demente* (the patient who has it) refer simply to cognitive ability, but Spanish speakers associate them with *locura* (insanity) and institutionalization in the *manicomio* (crazy house)—unimaginably degrading prospects in a culture that venerates its elders. *La chochera*, meaning "a state of diminished or lost mental faculties," is much less emotionally charged. Also used to describe an overly doting grandma, it is a much gentler way to deliver a devastating diagnosis.

What's the Diagnosis?

acne	acné	ahl NEH
AIDS	SIDA	SEE thah
allergies	alergias	ah LEHR hyahs
Alzheimer's	la enfermedad de Alzheimer	lah_ehn fehr meh THAHTH theh_AHLS hay mehr
angina	angina	ahn HEE nah
appendicitis	apendicitis	ah pehn dee SEE tees
arteriosclerosis	arteriosclerosis	ahr teh ryohs kleh ROH sees
arthritis	artritis	ahr TREE tees
asthma	asma	AHS mah
broken bone	un hueso fracturado	oon WEH soh

bronchitis	bronquitis	brohn KEE tees
cancer	cáncer	KAHN sehr
cataracts	cataratas	kah tah RAH tahs
cholera	cólera	KOH leh rah
cirrhosis	cirrosis	see RROH sees
cold	catarro	kah TAH rroh
colic	cólico	KOH lee koh
coronary artery disease (CAD)	enfermedad de las arterias coronarias	ehn fehr meh THAHTH theh lahs ahr THE ryahs koh roh NAH ryahs
dementia	pérdida de facultades mentales	PEHR thee thah theh fah kool TAH thehs mehn TAH lehs
diabetes	diabetes	dyah BEH tehs
diarrhea	diarrea	dyah RREH_ah
ear infection	una infección del oído	OO nah_een fehk SYOHN dehl oh EE thoh
emphysema	enfisema	ehn fee SEH mah
epilepsy	epilepsia	eh pee LEHP syah
fibromyalgia	fibromialgia	fee vroh MYAHL hyah
gallstones	cálculos biliares	KAHL koo lohs bee LYAH rehs
gastroesophageal reflux disease (GERD)	gastroesofagitis	gahs troh_eh soh fah HEE tees
glaucoma	glaucoma	glaw KOH mah
gonorrhea	gonorrea	goh noh RREH_ah

continues

What's the Diagnosis? (continued)

gout	gota	GOH tah
hay fever	fiebre del heno	FYEH vreh thehl EH noh
headache	dolor de cabeza	doh LOHR theh kah VEH sah
heart attack	ataque cardíaco	ah TAH keh kahr THEE_ah koh
hemorrhoids	almorranas	ahl moh RRAH nahs
hepatitis	hepatitis	eh pah TEE tees
herpes	herpe(s) (S is optional.)	EHR peh(s)
high blood pressure	presión (tensión) arterial	preh SYOHN (tehn SYOHN) ahr teh RYAHL
HIV	VIH/virus de inmunodefici- encia humano	beh_ee_hache/ BEE roos theh_een moo noh deh fee SYEHN syah
hives	ronchas	RROHN chahs
irritable bowel syndrome (IBS)	síndrome del intestino irritable	SEEN droh meh thehl een tehs TEE noh_ee rree TAH vleh
incontinence	incontinencia	een kohn tee NEHN syah
bowel ...	... fecal	feh KAHL
bladder ...	... urinaria	oo ree NAH ryah
influenza (regional variations)	gripe/gripa	GREE peh/ GREE pah

joint separation	separación de la articulación	seh pah rah SYOHN deh lah_ahr tee koo lah SYOHN
kidney stone	piedra/ cálculo renal	PYEH thrah/KAHL koo loh rreh NAHL
leukemia	leucemia	lew SEH myah
lupus	lupus	LOO poos
malnourishment	malnutrición	mahl noo tree SYOHN
measles	sarampión	sah rahm PYOHN
meningitis	meningitis	meh neen HEE tees
migraine	jaqueca	hah KEH kah
mumps	paperas	pah PEH rahs
osteoarthritis	osteoartritis	ohs teh_oh_ahr TREE tees
osteoporosis	osteoporosis	ohs teh_oh poh REE sees
overdose	sobredosis	soh vreh THOH sees
paralysis	parálisis	pah RAH lee sees
Parkinson's disease	la enfermedad de Parkinson	lah ehn fehr meh THAHTH theh PAHR keen sohn
pneumonia	pulmonía/ neumonía	pool moh NEE AH/ new moh NEE_ah
poisoning	envenenammiento	ehm beh neh nah MYEHN toh
rheumatoid arthritis	artritis reumatoide	ahr TREE tees rew mah TOY theh
sinusitis	sinusitis	see noo SEE tees
sprain	torcedura/ esguince	tohr seh THOO rah/ ehs GEEN she
strep throat	una infección estreptocócica	OO na_een fehk SYOHN ehs trehp toh KOH see kah

continues

What's the Diagnosis? (continued)

stroke	una embolia cerebral	OO nah_ehm BOH lyah seh reh VRAHL
syphilis	sífilis	SEE fee lees
tetanus	tétano	TEH tah noh
tinnitus	un zumbido en el oído	oon soom BEE thoh_ehn ehl oh EE thoh
tonsilitis	amigdalitis	ah meeg dah LEE tees
ulcer	úlcera	OOL seh rah
whooping cough	tos ferina	tohs feh REE nah
yeast infection	una infección de hongos	OO nah_een fehk SYOHN deh OHN gohs

¡Ojo!

Don't forget the common cold. Here are just three of the many ways to say "Do you have a cold?" in Spanish. Other regional variations are easily recognizable:

¿Tiene resfrío?	TYEH neh rrehs FREE oh
¿Tiene catarro?	TYEH neh kah TAH rroh
¿Está resfriado?	ehs TAH rrehs free AH thoh

Seeing a Specialist

After the diagnosis has been made, the patient may need to see a specialist or receive other services. Here's how to indicate the right ones. Note that many Spanish words for specialties are highly similar to their English equivalents:

[...] need(s) to see a/an ...
[...] necesita ver a ...
[...] neh seh SEE tah vehr ah ...

anesthesiologist	un anestesista	oon ah nehs teh TEES tah
cardiologist	un cardiólogo	oon kahr THYOH loh goh
chiropractor	un quiropráctico	oon kee roh PRAHK tee koh
dermatologist	un dermatólogo	oon dehr mah TOH lo go
gastroenter-ologist	un gastroenteró-logo	oon gahs troh_ehn teh ROH loh goh
gynecologist	un ginecólogo	oon hee neh KOH loh go
neurologist	un neurólogo	oon new ROH loh goh
nurse practitioner	una enfermera capacitada	OO nah_ehn fehr MEH rah kah pah see TAH thah
obstetrician	un obstetra	oon ohvs TEH trah
occupational therapist	un terapeuta	oon teh rah PEW tah
oncologist	un oncólogo	oon ohn KOH loh goh

continues

continued

ophthalmologist	un oftalmálogo	oon ohf tahl MOH loh goh
optometrist	un optometrista	oon ohp toh meh TREES tah
orthodontist	un ortodoncista	oon ohr toh thohn SEES tah
orthopedist	un ortopédico	oon ohr toh PEH thee koh
pathologist	un patólogo	oon pah TOH loh goh
pediatrician	un pediatra	oon peh DYAH trah
physical therapist	un terapeuta	oon teh rah PEW tah
podiatrist	un podiatra	oon poh THYAH trah
proctologist	un proctólogo	oon prohk TOH loh goh
psychiatrist	un psiquiatra	oon see KYAH trah
psychologist	un psicólogo	oon see KOH loh goh
radiologist	un radiólogo	oon rrah THYOH loh goh
social worker	un trabajador social	oon trah vah hah THOHR soh SYAHL
surgeon	un cirujano	oon see roo HAH noh
urologist	un urólogo	oon oo ROH loh goh
vascular surgeon	un cirujano vascular	oon see roo HAH noh vahs koo LAHR

Cancer

When cancer is the diagnosis, you'll need some special words to explain it. Here are some of the most useful:

We found …
Encontramos …
ehn kohn TRAH mohs

an abnormality	una anormalidad	OO na_ah nohr mah lee THAHTH
a cyst	un quiste	oon KEES teh
a lesion	una llaga	OO nah YAH gah
a lump	un bulto	oom BOOL toh
a shadow	una opacidad	OO nah oh pah see THAHTH
a tumor	un tumor	oon too MOHR

The cells …
Las células …
lahs SEH loo lahs

are normal	son normales	sohn nohr MAH lehs
are benign	son benignas	sohm beh NEEG nahs
are malignant	son malignas	sohm mah LEEG nahs
grow very fast	crecen rápidamente	kreh sehn RRAH pee thah MEHN teh

HIV/AIDS

HIV and AIDS are very serious diagnoses. The phrases in this section will let you offer crucial information, in their own language, to your Spanish-speaking patients. For phrases about treatment and preventing transmission of HIV, see Chapter 8.

AIDS is an infection caused by a virus called HIV.
SIDA es una infección causada por VIH, el virus de inmunodeficiencia humano.
SEE thah ehs OO nah_een fehk SYOHN kow SAH thah pohr veh ee AH cheh, ehl VEE roos theh_een moo noh theh fee SYEHN syah oo MAH noh

Once you are infected, you are HIV positive.
Después de infectarse, sus pruebas indican estado positivo.
dehs PWEHS theh_een fehk TAHR seh, soos PRWEH vahs een DEE kahn ehs TAH thoh poh see TEE voh

HIV attacks the body's ability to fight infections, even minor ones like a cold.
El VIH ataca su habilidad de superar hasta la menor infección como un catarro.
ehl veh ee AH cheh_ah TAH kah soo ah vee lee THAHTH theh soo peh RAHR AHS tah lah meh NOHR een fehk SYOHN KOH moh_oon kah TAH rroh

You can be HIV positive for many years before you actually become ill with AIDS.

Puede tener una infección positiva del VIH por muchos años antes de enfermarse sintomáticamente con SIDA.

PWEH theh teh NEHR OO nah_een fehk SYOHM poh see TEE vah thehl veh ee AH cheh_AHN tehs theh_ehn fehr MAHR seh seen toh MAH tee kah MEHN teh kohn SEE thah

There is no known cure for AIDS yet, but there are treatments that can help keep you well and prolong your life.

Hasta ahora el SIDA es incurable, pero existen tratamientos para aliviar sus síntomas y extender su vida.

AHS tah_ah OH rah_ehl SEE thah_ehs een koo RAH vleh, PEH roh ehk SEES tehn trah tah MYEHN tohs PAH rah_ah lee VYAHR soos SEEN toh mahs ee ehs tehn DEHR soo VEE thah

HIV is transmitted through sexual contact, blood, breastfeeding, and from a pregnant woman to her fetus.

El VIH se transmite por contacto sexual, por la sangre, por dar el pecho, y también una madre se lo puede pasar al feto en el vientre.

ehl veh ee_AH cheh seh trahns MEE teh pohr kohn TAHK toh sehk SWAHL, pohr la SAHN greh, pohr thahr ehl PEH choh, ee tahm BYEHN OO na MAH threh seh loh PWEH theh pah SAHR ahl FEH toh ehn ehl VYEHN treh

Both women and men can be infected and spread the disease through any type of sexual contact.

Los dos sexos pueden ser infectados y luego infectar a otros por cualquier forma de contacto sexual.

lohs thohs SEHK sohs PWEH thehn sehr een fehk TAH thohs ee LWEH goh_een fehk TAHR ah_OH trohs pohr kwahl KYEHR FOHR mah theh kohn TAHK toh sehk SWAHL

You can also get it from sharing needles with an infected person.

También puede contaminarse usando las jeringas infectadas de otra persona.

tahm BYEHN PWEH theh kohn tah mee NAHR seh_oo SAHN doh lahs heh REEN gahs een fehk TAH thahs theh_OH trah pehr SOH nah

Chapter 8

Treatment

In discussing treatment plans with your Hispanic patients, you'll need more than vocabulary. You'll also need an understanding of the beliefs and ideas they hold about medications and modes of healing that may be unfamiliar to you. It's vital they understand you, but to ensure a good outcome, it's vital you first understand *them*.

This chapter gives you both the language you want and the cultural insight you need to give your Hispanic patients the best possible care.

What Else Are You Taking?

Among many Latinos, especially those from Mexico, Central America, and the Caribbean, there is a long tradition of consulting a traditional healer, *un curandero*, for treatment of health problems. That person, although skilled and knowledgeable, is unlicensed, and may be prescribing treatments from an herbal medicine shop, *una botánica*. To prevent harmful interactions, it's important that you know if the patient is already treating his or her problem in some other way:

Are you consulting any other person for treatment of this condition?

¿Consulta con otra persona para tratar esta condición?

kohn SOOL tah kohn OH trah pehr SOH nah PAH rah trah TAHR EHS tah kohn dee SYOHN

What treatment has he/she ordered for you?

¿Qué tratamiento le ha mandado hacer?

keh trah tah MYEHN toh leh_ah mahn DAH thoh_ah SEHR

Are you taking any herbs or other natural remedies?

¿Toma usted hierbas u otros remedios naturales?

TOH mah_oos TEHTH YEHR vahs ooh_OH trohs rreh MEH thyohs nah too RAH lehs

Can you write down for me the names of the herbs/preparations?

¿Puede escribirme los nombres de las hierbas/preparaciones?

PWEH theh_ehs kree BEER meh lohs NOHM brehs theh lahs YEHR vahs /preh pah rah SYOH nehs

What you are currently doing ____ [insert from below] this treatment.

Eso que está haciendo […] nuestro tratamiento.

EH soh keh_ehs TAH_ah SYEHN doh […] NWEHS troh trah tah MYEHN toh

> will help
> ayuda con
> ah YOO thah kohn

> will interfere with
> interfiere con
> een tehr FYEH reh kohn

will defeat
niega los efectos de
NYEH gah lohs eh FEHK tohs theh

will have dangerous/unpleasant side effects for
le causará efectos colaterales peligrosos
(desagradables)
leh kow sah RAH eh FEHK tohs coh lah teh
RAH lehs peh lee GROH sohs (deh sah grah
THAH vlehs)

For the success of this treatment plan, I must ask
you to discontinue all other treatments.
Para el éxito de este plan de tratamiento, tengo que
pedirle que deje de utilizar todo tratamiento ajeno.
PAH rah_ehl EHK see toh theh_EHS teh plahn
deh trah tah MYEHN toh, TEHN goh keh peh
THEER leh keh DEH heh theh_oo tee lee SAHR
TOH thoh trah tah MYEHN toh_ah HEH noh

Over-the-Counter Options

Many simple remedies can help your patients. Here
are some words for things your patients can find at
the drugstore. To make the suggestion, start by saying the following:

You should get ...
Debe conseguir ...
DEH veh kohn seh GEER

You can use ...
Puede usar ...
PWEH theh_oo SAHR

With either of these lead-ins, it is not always necessary to include an article ("the" or "a").

adhesive tape	cinta adhesiva	SEEN tah_ah theh SEE vah
bandage	una venda	OO nah VEHN dah
Band-Aid	una curita	OO nah koo REE tah
cane	un bastón	oom bahs TOHN
cough syrup	un jarabe para la tos	oon hah RAH veh PAH rah lah tohs
creams	cremas	KREH mahs
crutches	muletas	moo LEH tahs
eye drops	gotas para los ojos	GOH tahs PAH rah lohs OH hohs
eye patch	un parche	oom PAHR cheh
gauze	gasa	GAH sah
hydrogen peroxide	agua oxigenada	AH gwah_ohk see heh NAH thah
ice pack	una bolsa de hielo	OO nah BOHL sah theh YEH loh
iodine	yodo	YOH thoh
laxative	un laxante	oon lahk SAHN teh
lozenges	pastillas	pahs TEE yahs
ointment	un ungüento	oon oon GWEHN toh
powder	talco	TAHL koh
sling	un cabestrillo	oon kah vehs TREE yoh
splint	una férula	OO nah FEH roo lah
	un soporte	oon soh POR teh

vitamins	vitaminas	vee tah MEE nahs
walker	una andadera	OO nah_ahn dah THEH rah
wheelchair	una silla de ruedas	OO na SEE yah theh RWEH thahs

Prescription Medications

In the Hispanic world, it is normal and legal for patients to self-medicate based solely on the advice of a licensed pharmacist. Patients simply describe a condition to the pharmacist, who then recommends and dispenses what would elsewhere be considered a controlled medication.

This frequently works, but occasionally there is trouble. Inevitably, there are misdiagnoses, and medication is dispensed inappropriately. Your patients know this, so many are wary of medicines and their use. If you're prescribing medication, gain your patients' confidence by using the vocabulary in this section to explain what it's for, how it will work, and the possible side effects. And stress the importance of following instructions to the letter:

It is extremely important to follow the instructions exactly as indicated.
Es importantísimo seguir las indicaciones al pie de la letra.
ehs eem pohr tahn TEE see moh seh GEER lahs eens trook SYOH nehs ahl pyeh theh lah LEH trah

Pharmaceutical Families

In the following list, the first Spanish word translates the English, but such words are not generally used by the public. The parenthetical phrase describes the medicine by its function, which is much more likely to be understood by Spanish speakers. Rather than "It is an analgesic," say "It reduces pain."

> This medication is [insert medicine name]
> Este medicamento es […]
> EHS teh meh thee kah MEHN toh_ehs
>
> This medication [insert parenthetical description]
> Este medicamento […]
> EHS teh meh thee kah MEHN toh

analgesic/ antipyretic (reduces pain and fever)	analgésico y antipirético (reduce dolor y fiebre)	ah nahl HEH see koh ee ahn tee pee REH tee koh (rreh THOO seh doh LOHR ee FYEH vreh)
antacid (relieves indigestion)	antiácido (calma la indigestión)	ahn TYAH see thoh (KAHL mah lah_een dee gehs TYOHN)
antiasthmatic (clears the bronchial tubes and lungs)	antiasmático (abre los bron- quios y pulmones)	ahn tee_ahs MAH tee koh (AH vreh lohs BROHN kyohs ee pool MOH nehs)
antibiotic (fights infection)	antibiótico (combate la infección)	ahn tee BYOH tee koh (kohm BAH teh lah–een fehk SYOHN)
anticoagulant (prevents formation of clots)	anticoagulante (impide la formación de coágulos)	ahn tee koh ah goo LAHN te (eem PEE theh lah fohr mah SYOHN deh koh AH goo lohs)

antiglycemic (lowers blood sugar)	antiglicémico (reduce la glucosa en la sangre)	ahn tee glee SEH mee koh (rreh THOO seh lah gloo KOH sah_ehn lah SAHN greh)
anti-inflammatory (reduces inflammation)	anti-inflamatorios (reduce la inflamación)	ahn tee een flah mah TOH ryohs (rreh THOO seh lah_een flah mah SYOHN)
anti-anxiety medication (lowers anxiety level)	anti-ansiedad (alivia la ansiedad)	ahn tee ahn syeh THAHTH (ah LEE vyah lah_ahn syeh THAHTH)
antidepressant (helps avoid depression)	antidepresivo (evita la depresión)	ahn tee theh preh SEE voh (eh VEE tah lah theh preh SYOHN)
anticonvulsant (helps avoid convulsions)	anticonvulsivo (evita convulsiones)	ahn tee kohm bool SEE voh (eh VEE tah kohm bool SYOH nehs)
anticholesterol medication (controls cholesterol levels)	anticolesterol (controla los lípidos en la sangre)	ahn tee koh lehs teh ROHL (kohn TROH lah lohs LEE pee thohs ehn lah SAHN greh)
antihistamine (relieves allergic reactions)	antihistamina (alivia reacciones alérgicas)	ahn tee_ees tah MEE nah (ah LEE vyah rreh ahk SYOH nehs ah LEHR hee kahs)

continues

continued

antihypertensive (controls high blood pressure)	antihipertensivo (controla la tensión arterial elevada)	ahn tee ee pehr tehn SEE voh (kohn TROH lah lah tehn SYOHN ahr teh RYAHL eh leh VAH thah)
antiviral (hinders viral activity)	antiviral (impide la acción de un virus)	ahn tee vee RAHL (eem PEE theh lah_ahk SYOHN deh_oom BEE roos)
diuretic (increases urine production)	diurético (provoca la producción de orina)	dyoo REH tee koh (proh VOH kah lah proh thook SYOHN theh_oh REE nah)
sedative (calms)	calmante (tranquiliza)	kahl MAHN teh (trahn kee LEE sah)
sleep aid (aids falling asleep)	somnífero (facilita el dormir)	sohm NEE feh roh (fah see LEE tah_ehl thohr MEER)
steroid (reduces inflammation)	esteroide (reduce inflamación)	ehs teh ROY theh (rreh THOO seh_een flah mah SYOHN)
stimulant (enhances physical or mental response)	estimulante (mejora la reacción física o mental)	ehs tee moo LAHN teh (meh HOH rah lah rreh ahk SYOHN FEE see kah_oh mehn TAHL)
vaccine (establishes immunity)	vacuna (establece inmunidad)	vah KOO nah (ehs tah VLEH seh_een moo nee THAHTH)

Rx: Questions and Instructions

The following words and phrases will help patients understand more about their prescriptions:

I'd like you to have this medication.
Quisiera recetarle este medicamento.
kee SYEH rah rreh seh TAHR leh_EHS teh meh
thee kah MEHN toh

Have you ever taken this medicine before?
¿Ha tomado esta medicina antes?
ah toh MAH thoh_EHS tah meh thee SEE
nah_AHN tehs

Did it help?
¿Le dio alivio?
leh thyoh_ah LEE vyoh

I am going to give you an injection.
Voy a ponerle una inyección.
boy ah poh NEHR leh_OO nah_een yehk SYOHN

This is a prescription for your medicine.
Esto es una receta para su medicina.
EHS toh_ehs OO nah reh SEH tah PAH rah soo
meh thee SEE nah

You can have it filled at any pharmacy.
Se la pueden hacer en cualquier farmacia.
seh lah PWEH thehn ah SEHR ehn kwahl
KYEHR fahr MAH syah

You need to take the medicine exactly as instructed.
Usted tiene que tomar la medicina exactamente
como está indicado.
oos TEHTH TYEH neh keh toh MAHR lah meh
thee SEE nah_ehk sahk tah MEHN teh KOH
moh_ehs TAH_een dee KAH thoh

Call me ...
Llámeme a mí ...
YAH meh meh_ah mee

> if you do not feel better in ___ days.
> si no se siente mejor dentro de ___ días.
> see noh seh SYEHN teh meh HOHR thehn
> troh theh ___ THEE ahs

> if you feel worse.
> si se siente peor.
> see seh SYEHN teh peh OHR

If you have any negative reactions ...
Si tiene cualquier reacción negativa ...
see TYEH neh kwahl KYEHR rreh ahk SYOHN
neh gah TEE vah

> stop the medicine at once and call me.
> deje de usarla y llámeme inmediatamente.
> DEH heh theh_oo SAHR lah ee YAH meh
> meh_een meh thyah tah MEHN teh

> Negative reactions might be ...
> Las posibles reacciones negativas son ...
> lahs poh SEE vlehs rreh_ahk SYOH nehs neh
> gah TEE vahs sohn ...

rash	ronchas	RROHN chahs
itching	picazón	pee kah SOHN
nausea	náuseas	NOW seh ahs
vomiting	vómitos	VOH mee tohs
diarrhea	diarrea	dyah RREH áh

You should start feeling better in _____ hours (days).
Comenzará a sentirse mejor dentro de _____ horas (días).
koh mehn sah RAH_ah sehn TEER seh meh HOHR THEHN troh theh _____ OH rahs (THEE ahs)

Finish all the medication, even if you feel better.
Hace falta acabar toda la medicina, aun cuando se sienta mejor.
AH seh FAHL tah_ah kah VAHR TOH thah lah meh thee SEE nah, own KWAN doh seh SYEHN tah meh HOHR

If you miss a dose, take it when you remember, ...
Si se le ovida una dósis, tómela cuando se dé cuenta, ...
see seh leh_ohl VEE thah_OO nah THOH sees, TOH meh lah KWAHN doh seh THEH KWEHN tah

    ... then get back on schedule.
    ... luego vuelva al horario de dosificación.
    LWEH goh VWEHL vah_ahl oh RAH ryoh theh thoh see fee kah SYOHN

Do not "double up" on doses.
No tome jamás dos dosis en una sola vez.
noh TOH meh hah MAHS dohs DOH sees ehn OO nah SOH lah vehs

Let's lower (increase) the dosage.
Reduzcamos (aumentemos) la dosis.
rreh thoos KAH mohs (ow mehn TEH mos) lah THOH sees

You need to …
Tiene que …
TYEH neh keh …

> measure it carefully.
> medirlo con cuidado.
> meh THEER loh kohn kwee THAH thoh
>
> read the label.
> leer la etiqueta.
> leh EHR lah_eh tee KEH tah
>
> refrigerate it.
> refrigerarlo.
> rreh free heh RAHR loh

(It's important to) take the medicine …
(Hace falta que) tome la medicina …
(AH seh FAHL tah keh) TOH meh lah meh thee
SEE nah

> with food
> con comida
> kohn koh MEE thah
>
> _____ hours after meals.
> _____ horas después de comer.
> _____ OH rahs thehs PWEHS theh koh
> MEHR
>
> _____ hours before meals.
> _____ horas antes de comer.
> _____ OH rahs AHN tehs theh koh MEHR
>
> between meals.
> entre las comidas.
> EHN treh lahs koh MEE thahs

when you have pain.
cuando tiene dolor.
KWAN doh TYEH neh thoh LOHR

with water.
con agua.
kohn AH gwah

____ times.
____ veces.
____ VEH sehs

every____ hours.
cada ____ horas.
KAH thah ____ OH rahs

Side Effects

This medicine may cause you to …
Es posible que este medicamento le provoque …
ehs poh SEE vleh keh_ehs teh meh thee kah
MEHN toh leh proh VOH keh

be drowsy.
el sueño.
ehl SWEH nyoh

have insomnia.
insomnia.
ees SOHM nyah

have blurred vision.
la vista nublada.
lah VEES tah noo VLAH thah

have a dry mouth.
sequedad de la boca.
seh keh THAHTH theh lah VOH kah

be nauseated.

náuseas.

NOW seh ahs

lose your appetite.

una falta de apetito.

OO nah FAHL tah theh_ah peh TEE toh

have diarrhea.

diarrhea.

dyah RREH ah

be constipated.

estreñimiento.

ehs treh nyee MYEHN toh

have a change in the color of your urine.

un cambio del color de la orina.

oon KAHM byoh thehl koh LOHR theh
lah_oh REE nah

have palpitations.

palpitaciones.

pahl pee tah SYOH nehs

have a rash.

ronchas / una erupción.

RROHN chahs / OO na_eh roop SYOHN

Beyond Medication

Sometimes more evaluation is needed, or the
patient's condition requires something other than
medication:

You need (to have) …
Necesita …
neh seh SEE tah

> more tests.
> más pruebas.
> mahs PRWEH vahs
>
> to be hospitalized …
> hospitalizarse …
> ohs pee tah lee SAHR seh
>
> have an operation.
> una operación.
> OO nah_oh peh rah SYOHN
>
> have a transfusion.
> una transfusión.
> OO nah trans foo SYOHN
>
> stay in bed.
> guardar cama.
> gwahr THAHR KAH mah
>
> eat more (less).
> comer más (menos).
> koh MEHR mahs (MEH nohs)
>
> maintain a special diet.
> seguir una dieta especial.
> seh GEER OO nah DYEH tah_ehs peh
> SYAHL
>
> drink more fluids.
> tomar más líquidos.
> toh MAHR mahs LEE kee thohs
>
> restrict your fluids.
> limitar sus líquidos.
> lee mee TAHR soos LEE kee thohs

limit use of your ___.
limitar su uso de ___.
lee mee TAHR soo_OO soh theh ___

exercise your ___.
hacer ejercicio con ___.
ah SEHR eh hehr SEE syoh kohn ___

keep your ___ elevated.
mantener elevado su ___.
mahn teh NEHR eh leh VAH thoh soo ___

avoid contact with___.
evitar contacto con ___.
eh vee TAHR kohn TAHK toh kohn ___

have a cast on your ___.
un yeso en su ___.
oon YEH soh_ehn soo ___

keep this dry.
mantener esto seco.
mahn teh NEHR SEH koh

stop smoking.
dejar de fumar.
theh HAHR theh foo MAHR

stop drinking alcohol.
dejar de tomar alcohol.
theh HAHR theh toh MAHR ahl koh_OHL

stop using drugs.
dejar de usar drogas.
theh HAHR theh_oo SAHR throh gahs

avoid straining when you defecate.
evitar forzarse cuando defeca.
eh vee TAHR fohr SAHR seh KWAHN doh
theh FEH kah

I want to see you again in _____.
Quiero que me vuelva a ver en _____.
KYEH roh keh meh BWEHL vah_ah vehr
ehn _____

Special Instructions for ...

Certain medical situations call for specialized vocabulary. This section contains important phrases you'll use to guide patients with particular needs.

Cancer

The best treatment for this kind of cancer is ...
El mejor tratamiento para este tipo de cáncer
es ...
ehl meh HOHR trah tah MYEHN toh PAH
rah_EHS teh TEE poh theh KAHN sehr ehs

chemotherapy	quimoterapia	kee moh teh RAH pyah
biological	biológico	byoh LOH hee koh
radiation	radiación	rrah dyah SYOHN
surgery	cirugía	see roo HEE ah

You may ...
Es posible que usted ...
ehs poh SEE vleh keh_oos TEHTH

feel weak and fatigued.
se sienta débil.
seh SYEHN tah THEH veel

have ...
experimente ...
ehks peh ree MEHN teh

> constipation.
> estreñimiento.
> ehs treh nyee MYEHN toh
>
> diarrhea.
> diarrea.
> dyah RREH ah
>
> nausea.
> náuseas.
> NOW seh ahs
>
> vomiting.
> vómitos.
> VOH mee tohs

become more susceptible to infection.
esté más susceptible a infectarse.
ehs TEH mahs soo sehp TEE vleh_ah_een
fehk TAHR seh

lose some or all of your hair.
se le caiga el pelo, parcial o totalmente.
seh leh KAY gah_ehl PEH loh, pahr SYAHL
oh toh tahl MEHN teh

have a change in your skin color.
el color de su piel cambie.
ehl koh LOHR theh soo pyehl KAHM byeh

become infertile.
no pueda concebir o procrear.
noh PWEH thah kon seh VEER oh proh kreh
AHR

lose or gain large amounts of weight.

experimente grandes aumentos o pérdidas de peso.

ehs peh ree MEHN teh GRAHN dehs ow MEHN tohs oh PEHR thee thahs theh PEH soh

Cardiorespiratory Problems

You must ...

Tiene que ...   TYEH neh keh

Necesita ...   neh seh SEE tah

Es necesario ...   ehs neh seh SAH ryoh

sleep with your head and shoulders elevated.

dormir con la cabeza y los hombros elevados.

dohr MEER kohn lah kah VEH sah ee lohs OHM brohs eh leh VAH thohs

avoid salty foods.

evitar la comida salada.

eh vee TAHR lah koh MEE thah sah LAH thah

You must not ...

Usted no debe ...

oos TEHTH noh THEH veh

overexert yourself.

esforzarse demasiado.

ehs fohr SAHR seh theh mah SYAH thoh

work outside in very cold weather.

trabajar afuera cuando hace mucho frío.

trah vah HAHR ah FWEH rah KWAHN doh_AH seh MOO choh FREE oh

You need to have oxygen.
Usted necesita oxígeno.
oos TEHTH neh seh SEE tah_ohk SEE heh noh

Do not turn up the oxygen past here.
No abra la llave del oxígeno más allá de aquí.
noh_AH vrah lah YAH veh thehl ohk SEE heh noh
mahs ah YAH deh_ah KEE

To use your inhaler:
Para usar su inhalador:
PAH rah_oo SAHR soo_een ah lah THOHR

> Shake it.
> Agítelo.
> ah HEE teh loh
>
> Inhale one puff.
> Aspire una atomización.
> ahs PEE reh_OO nah_ah toh mee sah
> SYOHN
>
> Hold your breath for as long as possible.
> Aguante el aliento lo más posible.
> ah GWAHN teh_ehl ah LYEHN toh loh
> mahs poh SEE vleh
>
> Wait 30 to 60 seconds.
> Espere desde treinta a sesenta segundos.
> ehs PEH reh THEHS theh TREYN
> tah_ah seh SEHN tah seh GOON dohs
>
> Then inhale the second puff ...
> Luego aspire la segunda atomización ...
> LWEH goh_ahs PEE reh lah seh GOON
> dah_ah toh mee sah SYOHN

... and hold it as long as possible.
... y aguántela lo más posible.
... ee ah GWAHN teh lah loh mahs poh SEE
vleh

Get an air conditioner if you can.
Utilice un acondicionador de aire si puede.
oo tee LEE seh_oon ah kohn dee syoh nah THOHR
theh_AY reh see PWEH theh

Stay inside on "bad air" days.
No salga de casa cuando se declaran días de alta con-
taminación.
noh SAL gah theh KAH sah KWAHN doh seh theh
KLAH rahn THEE ahs theh_AHL tah kohn tah mee
nah SYOHN

Take your pulse every day before taking your medicine.
Tómese el pulso cada día antes de tomar su medicina.
TOH meh seh_ehl POOL soh KAH thah THEE
ah_AHN tehs theh toh MAHR soo meh thee SEE nah

If your pulse is below ____, do not take your digoxin.
Si su pulso es menos de ____, no tome su digoxin.
see soo POOL soh_ehs MEH nohs theh ____, noh
TOH meh soo digoxin

If you have angina, put a nitroglycerin tab (or spray)
under your tongue.
Si sufre una angina, coloque una pastilla (o una atomización) de Nitroglicerina debajo de la lengua.
see SOO freh OO nah_ahn HEE nah, koh LOH
keh_OO nah pahs TEE yah_(oh_OO nah_ah toh
mee sah SYOHN) theh NEE troh glee SEH REE
nah theh VAH hoh theh lah LEHN gwah

Take your water pill every day.
Tome su medicina diurética todos los días.
TOH meh soo meh thee SEE nah dyoo REH tee
kah TOH thohs lohs THEE ahs

You can continue (resume) your sexual activities.
Puede continuar con (reanudar) sus actividades
sexuales.
PWEH theh kohn tee NWAHR kohn (reh ah noo
THAHR) soos ahk tee vee THAH thehs sehk
SWAH lehs

Cardiovascular Problems

Take your blood pressure every day.
Tómese la tensión arterial todos los días.
TOH meh seh lah tehn SYOHN ahr teh RYAHL
TOH thohs lohs THEE ahs

If your pressure is lower than _____, do not take your
blood pressure medication.
Si tiene la tensión inferior a _____, no tome su medicina hipertensiva.
see TYEH neh lah tehn SYOHN een feh RYOHR
ah _____, noh TOH meh soo meh thee SEE nah_ee
pehr tehn SEE vah

If it is higher than _____, take your blood pressure
medication.
Si la tiene más alta que _____, tome su medicina
hipertensiva.
see lah TYEH neh mahs AHL tah keh _____, TOH
meh soo meh thee SEE nah_ee pehr tehn SEE vah

You must take your blood pressure medication every
day ...
Tiene que tomar su medicina hipertensiva todos los
días ...
TYEH neh keh toh MAHR soo meh thee SEE nah
ee pehr tehn SEE vah TOH thohs lohs THEE ahs

> ... or you could have a heart attack or a stroke.
> ... ya que el fallar puede ocasionarle un ataque
> cardíaco o una embolia.
> yah keh_ehl fah YAHR PWEH theh_oh kah
> syoh NAHR leh_oon ah TAH keh kahr THEE
> ah koh_oh_OO nah_ehm BOH lyah

Check your pulse every day.
Tómese el pulso cada día.
TOH meh seh_ehl POOL soh KAH thah THEE ah

If it is less than _____, do not take your digoxin that
day.
Si es menos de _____, no tome su digoxin ese día.
see_ehs MEH nohs theh _____, noh TOH meh soo
digoxin EH seh THEE ah

Elevate your feet whenever possible.
Eleve los pies cuando pueda.
eh LEH veh lohs PYEHS KWAHN doh PWEH thah

You are on medication that thins your blood.
Usted está tomando una medicina que diluye su sangre.
oos TEHTH ehs TAH toh MAHN doh_OO nah meh
thee SEE nah keh thee LOO yeh soo SAHN greh

You may notice that you bruise easily,
Quizá note que se amorata más fácilmente,
kee SAH NOH teh keh seh_ah moh RAH tah mahs
FAH seel MEHN teh,

... and that your gums bleed.

... y que le sangran las encías.

ee keh leh SAHN grahn lahs ehn SEE ahs

If you experience any problems or anything out of the ordinary, call me, or call 9-1-1.

Si tiene cualquier problema o experimenta algo inesperado, llámeme, o llame al nueve uno uno.

see TYEH neh kwahl KYEHR proh VLEH mah_oh ehs peh ree MEHN tah AHL goh een ehs peh RAH thoh, YAH meh meh, oh YAH meh_ahl NWEH veh_OO noh_OO noh

Diabetes

Always carry ...

Siempre lleve consigo ...

SYEHM preh YEH veh kohn SEE goh ...

> your diabetic ID card.
>
> su tarjeta de diabético.
>
> soo tahr HEH tah theh thyah VEH tee koh
>
> candies.
>
> dulces.
>
> THOOL sehs

You need an insulin pump.

Usted necesita una dosificadora de insulina.

oos TEHTH neh seh SEE tah_OO nah thoh see fee kah THOH rah theh_een soo LEE nah

You need to test your blood sugar with this
machine at the prescribed times.
Necesita determinar su nivel de glucosa con este
aparato a las horas prescritas.
neh seh SEE tah theh tehr mee NAHR soo nee
VEHL theh gloo KOH sah kohn EHS teh_ah pah
RAH toh_ah lahs OH rahs prehs KREE tahs

If you …
Si usted …
see oos TEHTH …

> do not have enough insulin,
> no tiene suficiente insulina,
> noh TYEH neh soo fee SYEHN teh_een soo
> LEE nah

> use too much insulin,
> usa demasiada insulina,
> OO sah theh mah SYAH thah_een soo LEE nah

> do not follow the proper diet,
> no sigue un régimen apropiado,
> noh SEE geh_oon RREH hee mehn ah proh
> PYAH thoh

> go too long without eating after taking your
> insulin,
> si pasa demasiado tiempo sin comer depués de
> tomar la insulina,
> see PAH sah theh mah SYAH thoh TYEHM
> poh seen koh MEHR thehs PWEHS theh toh
> MAHR lah_een soo LEE nah

> exercise too much,
> hace ejercicio excesivo,
> AH seh eh hehr SEE syoh_ehk seh SEE voh

work too much,
trabaja demasiado,
trah VAH hah theh mah SYAH thoh

you may experience any of the following:
puede experimentar cualquiera de estos síntomas.
PWEH theh ehs peh ree mehn TAHR kwahl
KYEH rah theh_EHS tohs SEEN toh mahs

confusion	confusión	kohn foo SYOHN
dizziness	mareos	mah REH ohs
irritability	irritabilidad	ee rree tah vee lee THAHTH
nervousness	agitación	ah hee tah SYOHN
excessive thirst	mucha sed	MOO chah seth
weakness	debilidad	theh vee lee THAHTH
deep breathing	respiración profunda	rrehs pee rah SYOHN proh FOON dah
rapid breathing	respiración acelerada	rrehs pee rah SYOHN ah seh leh RAH thah
fainting	desmayos	thehs MAH yohs
hunger	hambre	AHM breh
nausea	náuseas	NOW seh ahs
headache	dolor de cabeza	thoh LOHR theh kah VEH sah
blurred vision	visión nublada	lah vee SYOHN noo VLAH thah
cold sweats	sudores fríos	soo THOH rehs FREE ohs
dry skin	piel seca	lah pyehl SEH kah
palpitations	palpitaciones	pahl pee tah SYOH nehs

| frequent urination | orinar con más frecuencia | oh ree NAHR kohn mahs freh KWEHN syah |
| vomit | vómitos | VOH mee tohs |

Then test your blood sugar.
Entonces pruebe su nivel de glucosa en la sangre.
ehn TOHN sehs prweh VEH soo nee VEHL theh
gloo KOH sah_ehn lah SAHN greh

Call the hospital emergency room.
Llame a la sala de emergencia.
YAH meh_ah lah SAH lah theh_eh mehr HEHN syah

If your blood sugar is low, drink some juice or eat
some candy.
Si su nivel de glucosa es bajo, tome jugo o coma dulces.
see soo nee VEHL theh gloo KOH sah_ehs VAH hoh,
TOH meh HOO goh_oh KOH mah THOOL sehs

Inspect your feet every day.
Inspecciónese los pies cada día.
eens pehk SYOH neh seh lohs pyehs KAH thah
THEE ah

Gastrointestinal Problems

Your condition (illness) can be treated with proper
diet and/or medication.
Su condición (enfermedad) puede ser tratada con una
dieta apropiada y/o medicinas.
soo kohn dee SYOHN (ehn fehr meh THAHTH)
PWEH theh sehr trah TAH thah kohn OO nah
THYEH tah_ah proh PYAH thah_ee oh meh thee
SEE nahs

You must sleep with your head and shoulders elevated.
Debe dormir con la cabeza y los hombros elevados.
Deh veh thohr MEER kohn lah kah VEH sah_ee lohs
OHM brohs eh leh VAH thohs

Do not take aspirin, because it will make your condition worse.
No tome aspirina, porque empeorará su condición.
noh TOH meh_ahs pee REE nah, POHR keh_ehm
peh oh rah RAH soo kohn dee SYOHN

You must avoid these foods ____.
Debe evitar estos alimentos ____.
DEH veh_eh vee TAHR EHS tohs ah lee MEHN
tohs.

Do not eat 2 to 3 hours before you go to bed.
No coma nada dos o tres horas antes de acostarse.
noh KOH mah NAH thah thohs oh trehs OH rahs
AHN tehs theh_ah kohs TAHR seh

You cannot tolerate dairy products.
Usted no tolera los productos lácteos.
oos TEHTH noh toh LEH rah lohs proh THOOK
tohs LAHK teh ohs

You must eat small, frequent meals.
Sus comidas deben ser pequeñas y frecuentes.
soos koh MEE thahs THEH vehn sehr peh KEH
nyahs ee freh KWEHN tehs

You must be fed through a tube.
Tendrá que alimentarse a través de un tubo.
tehn DRAH keh_ah lee mehn TAHR seh_ah trah
VEHS theh_oon TOO voh

You must avoid liquids with your meals.
Debe evitar líquidos con sus comidas.
Deh veh_eh vee TAHR LEE kee thohs kohn soos
koh MEE thahs

Antacids will help your problem.
Aliviarán su problema los antiácidos.
ah lee vyah RAHN soo proh VLEH mah lohs ahn
TYAH see thohs

HIV/AIDS

You must be careful not to infect your sexual partner
with HIV.
Tiene que cuidar de no infectar a su pareja con el VIH.
TYEH neh keh kwee THAHR theh noh_een fehk
TAHR ah soo pah REH hah kohn ehl veh ee AH cheh

You should tell your mate (or any sex partner) that
you are HIV positive.
Tiene que decirle a su pareja que usted es "positivo,"
que definitivamente lleva el VIH.
TYEH neh keh theh SEER leh_ah soo pah REH
hah keh_oos TEHTH ehs poh see TEE voh, keh
theh fee nee tee vah MEHN teh YEH vah_ehl ve ee
AH cheh

If you don't tell them and you infect them, you could
be charged with a crime.
Si no se lo revela y luego le pasa la infección, se le
puede acusar de un crimen.
see noh seh loh rreh VEH lah ee LWEH goh leh
PAH sah lah_een fehk SYOHN, seh leh PWEH theh
ah koo SAHR theh oon KREE mehn

You must *always* use a condom when having any type of sexual contact.

Tiene que usar un condón *siempre* durante el coito.

TYEH neh keh_oo SAHR oon kohn DOHN SYEHM preh doo RAHN teh_ehl KOY toh

If your family and friends do not come into direct contact with your blood, semen, or vaginal secretions, they will not become infected.

Su familia y familiares no corren ningún riesgo de infectarse si no se contaminan con la infección por contacto directo con su sangre, su semen o sus secreciones vaginales.

soo fah MEE lyah ee fah mee LYAH rehs noh KOH rrehn neen GOON RRYEHS goh theh_een fehk TAHR seh see noh seh kohn tah MEE nahn kohn lah_een fehk SYOHN pohr kohn TAHK toh thee REHK toh kohn soo SAN greh, soo SEH mehn oh soos seh kreh SYOH nehs vah hee NAH lehs

You cannot spread this infection by kissing, sneezing, coughing, or sharing utensils.

Esta infección no se transmite por besos, estornudos, tos, o por compartir los cubiertos de la mesa.

EHS tah_een fehk SYOHN noh seh trahns MEE teh pohr VEH sohs, ehs tohr NOO thohs, tohs oh pohr kohm pahr TEER lohs koo VYEHR tohs theh lah MEH sah

The virus is not in sweat, urine, or feces, *only* blood, semen, vaginal secretions, and breast milk.

El virus no se encuentra en el sudor, la orina, o el excremento; se encuentra *sólo* en la sangre, el semen, las secreciones vaginales, y la leche del pecho.

ehl VEE roos noh seh_ehn KWEHN trah_ehn ehl
soo THOHR, lah_oh REE nah, oh_ehl ehks kreh
MEHN toh; she_ehn KWEHN trah SOH loh_ehn
lah SAHN greh, ehl SEH mehn, lahs seh kreh
SYOH nehs vah hee NAH lehs ee lah LEH cheh
thehl PEH choh

You can get it if infected blood gets in your eyes or
mouth, or into your body through a cut, scratch, or
other wound.

Usted puede infectarse si la sangre infectada entra en
su cuerpo por los ojos, la boca, o por una cortada, un
rasguño, o cualquier otra herida.

oos TEHTH PWEH theh_een fehk TAHR seh see
lah SAHN greh_een fehk TAH thah_EHN trah_ehn
soo KWEHR poh pohr lohs OH hohs, lah VOH
kah, oh pohr OO na kohr TAH thah, oon rrahs GOO
nyoh_oh kwahl KYEHR OH trah_eh REE thah

You must take your medications *exactly* as directed,
on time, several times a day.

Tiene que tomar las medicinas *exactamente* como están
recetadas, a las horas indicadas, varias veces al día.

TYEH neh keh toh MAHR lahs meh thee SEE nahs
ehk sahk tah MEHN teh KOH moh ehs TAHN reh
seh TAH thahs, ah lahs OH rahs een dee KAH thahs,
VAH ryahs VEH sehs ahl THEE ah

Avoid crowds and close contact with anyone who
is ill.

Evite la muchedumbre y el contacto con personas
enfermas.

eh VEE teh lah moo cheh THOOM breh_ee_ehl
kohn TAHK toh kohn pehr SOH nahs ehn FEHR
mahs

Muscular/Skeletal Problems

You need an ACE wrap.
Necesita una venda elástica *ACE*.
neh seh SEE tah_OO nah VEHN dah_eh LAHS tee kah *ACE*

It should be medium tight to reduce swelling.
Debe llevarla algo ajustada para que reduzca la hinchazón.
DEH veh yeh VAHR lah_AHL goh_ah hoos TAH thah PAH rah keh rreh DOOS kah lah_een chah SOHN

If it's too tight, it will cut off circulation.
Si aprieta demasiado, cortará la circulación de la sangre.
see_ah PRYEH tah theh mah SYAH thoh, kohr tah RAH lah seer koo lah SYOHN

If it's too loose, it will not be effective.
Si está demasiado floja, no sirve para nada.
see_ehs TAH theh mah SYAH thoh FLOH hah, noh SEER veh PAH rah NAH thah

Adjust it several times a day.
Ajústela varias veces al día.
ah HOOS teh lah VAH ryahs VEH sehs ahl THEE ah

Keep it elevated.
Manténgalo elevado.
mahn TEHN gah loh_eh leh VAH thoh

Use a cold pack to reduce pain—20 minutes on, 20 minutes off.
Póngale una bolsa fría por veinte minutos para reducir el dolor—luego quítesela por otros veinte minutos.

POHN gah leh_OO nah BOHL sah FREE ah pohr
VEYN teh mee NOO tohs PAH rah rreh thoo SEER
ehl thoh LOHR, LWEH goh KEE teh seh lah pohr
OH trohs VEYN teh mee NOO tohs

Don't put a cold pack directly on your skin.
No coloque una bolsa fría en contacto directo con la
piel.
noh koh LOH keh OO nah BOHL sah FREE ah ehn
kohn TAHK toh thee REHK toh kohn lah pyehl

If you don't have a cold pack, ...
Si no tiene una bolsa fría.
see noh TYEH neh_OO nah BOHL sah FREE
ah, ...

   ... a bag of frozen vegetables can be used for a
   cold pack.
   ... puede usar una bolsa de verduras congeladas
   en lugar de una bolsa fría.
   ... PWEH theh_oo SAHR OO nah BOHL sah
   theh vehr THOO rahs kohn heh LAH thahs
   ehn loo GAHR theh_OO nah BOHL sah FREE
   ah

Apply a warm/moist pack to relax muscles and
increase circulation.
Aplíquese una compresa tibia y húmeda para relajar
los músculos y estimular la circulación.
ah PLEE keh seh_OO nah kohm PREH sah TEE
vyah ee_OO meh thah PAH rah rreh lah HAHR
lohs MOOS koo lohs ee_ehs tee moo LAHR lah
seer koo lah SYOHN

Use crutches until I see you again.
Utilice las muletas hasta que usted vuelva a verme.
oo tee LEE seh lahs moo LEH tahs AHS tah keh
oos TEHTH VWEHL vah_ah VEHR meh

Don't use your ___ until I see you again.
No utilice su ___ hasta que usted vuelva a verme.
noh_oo tee LEE seh soo ___ AHS tah keh oos
TEHTH VWEHL vah_ah VEHR meh

Newborns

Newborn babies …
Los bebés recién nacidos …
lohs veh VEHS rreh SYEHN nah SEE thohs …

> must eat several times a day.
> deben comer varias veces al día.
> THEH vehn koh MEHR VAH ryahs VEH sehs
> ahl THEE ah
>
> usually eat every 2 or 3 hours.
> suelen comer cada dos o tres horas.
> SWEH lehn koh MEHR KAH thah thohs oh
> trehs OH rahs
>
> urinate approximately 8 to 10 times a day.
> orinan unas ocho a diez veces al día.
> oh REE nahn OO nahs OH choh ah dyehs
> VEH sehs ahl THEE ah
>
> have 2 to 4 bowel movements a day.
> defecan unas dos a cuatro veces al día.
> theh FEH kahn OO nas thohs ah KWAH troh
> VEH sehs ahl THEE ah

Do not give the baby solid food until the doctor
tells you it is okay.
No le dé alimentos sólidos al bebé hasta que el
médico se lo autorice.
noh leh theh_ah lee MEHN tohs SOH lee thohs ahl
veh VEH_AHS tah keh_ehl MEH thee koh seh
loh_ow toh REE seh

Always support the baby's head.
Apóyele siempre la cabeza al bebé.
ah POH yeh leh SYEHM preh lah kah VEH
sah_ahl veh VEH

You will need a pediatrician.
Va a necesitar a un pediatra.
bah_ah neh seh see TAHR ah_oon peh THYAH trah

Wound Care

You need to watch out for infection.
Vea que no se infecte su herida.
VEH ah keh noh seh_een FEHK teh soo_eh REE
thah

The signs of infection can be ...
Las indicaciones de una infección incluyen ...
lahs een dee kah SYOH nehs theh_OO nah_een
fehk SYOHN een KLOO yehn

> fever.
> fiebre.
> FYEH vreh

increased redness, heat, throbbing, pain, and swelling around the wound.

más enrojecimiento, calor, pulsación, dolor, e hinchazón en la región de la herida.

mahs ehn roh heh see MYEHN toh kah LOHR pool sah SYOHN doh LOHR eh_een chah SOHN ehn lah rreh HYOHN theh lah_eh REE thah

purulent drainage (pus) that has a foul odor.

secreción de pus maloliente.

seh kreh SYOHN theh poos mah loh LYEHN teh

If you get the bandage wet, change it.

Si la venda se moja, cámbiela.

see lah VEHN dah seh MOH hah, KAHM byeh lah

Discard the dirty bandage in a safe place where children and pets cannot reach it.

Deseche la venda sucia en un lugar seguro inaccesible a los niños y los animales.

deh SEH cheh lah VEHN dah SOO syah_ehn oon loo GAHR seh GOO roh_ee nahk seh SEE vleh_ah lohs NEE nyohs ee lohs ah nee MAH lehs

Always wash your hands before and after changing the bandage.

Lávese siempre las manos antes y después de cambiar la venda.

LAH veh seh SYEHM preh lahs MAH nohs AHN tehs ee thehs PWEHS theh kahm BYAHR lah VEHN dah

Hospitalization and Surgery

No matter what it's for, hospitalization takes the patient out of his or her element. For the patient who speaks only Spanish, almost everything about a hospital stay is disconcerting. There is the potential for getting lost, the anxiety about what comes next, the lack of familiar foods and entertainments, and— most of all—the separation from family and friends.

To a certain degree, patients will look to you for the support they would normally receive from those close to them. Using the words and phrases in this chapter, you can provide that. You'll be able to allay their concerns with information and reassurance. You'll also be able to communicate clearly about matters purely medical—surgery, medications, doctors' orders, and nursing care.

Communication—on many levels—is crucial to good hospital care. It starts with orienting patients and their families to this temporary "home."

Where Is the ...?

Most hospitals are big, busy places. Patients and visitors alike need help finding their way around, especially if they can't read the signs. You can assist Spanish speakers using the phrases and words that follow:

To locate a single thing:

> The _____ is that way.
> El/La _____ está por ahí.
> ehl (lah) _____ ehs TAH pohr ah_EE

To locate several things:

> The _____ are that way.
> Los/Las _____ están por ahí.
> ehl (lah) _____ ehs TAHN pohr ah_EE

It's ...
Está ...
ehs TAH

> down the hall.
> más adelante por el pasillo.
> mahs ah theh LAHN teh pohr ehl pah SEE yoh

> on the right.
> a la derecha.
> ah lah theh REH chah

> on the left.
> a la izquierda.
> ah lah_ees KYEHR thah

on the floor above (below).
en el piso arriba (abajo).
ehn ehl PEE soh_ah RREE vah (_ah VAH hoh)

Use these location names to help patients find their way:

administration	la administración	lah_ahth mee nees trah SYOHN
cafeteria	la cafetería	lah kah feh teh REE ah
cashier	el cajero	ehl kah HEH roh
chapel	la capilla	lah kah PEE yah
delivery room	la sala de partos	lah SAH lah theh PAHR tohs
elevator	el ascensor	ehl ah sehn SOHR
emergency room	la sala de emergencia	lah SAH lah theh_eh mehr HEHN syah
entrance	la entrada	lah_ehn TRAH thah
exit	la salida	lah sah LEE thah
gift shop	la tienda de regalos	lah TYEHN dah theh rreh GAH lohs
intensive care	la sala de cuidados intensivos	lah SAH lah theh kwee THAH thohs een tehn SEE vohs
laboratory	el laboratorio	ehl lah voh rah TOH ryoh
main lobby	el salón principal	ehl sah LOHM preen see PAHL
maternity ward	la sala de maternidad	lah SAH lah theh mah tehr nee THAHTH

continues

continued

nursery	la guardería (infantil)	lah gwahr theh REE ah (een fahn TEEL)
operating room	la sala de operaciones	lah SAH lah theh_oh peh rah SYOH nehs
radiology department	el departamento de radiología	ehl theh pahr tah MEHN toh theh rrah thyoh loh HEE ah
recovery room	la sala de recuperación	lah SAH lah theh rreh koo peh rah SYOHN
stairs	las escaleras	lahs ehs kah LEH rahs
telephone	el teléfono	ehl teh LEH foh noh
toilet	el baño	ehl VAH nyoh
waiting room	la sala de espera	lah SAH lah theh_ehs PEH rah
water fountain	la fuente de agua	lah FWEHN teh theh_AH gwah

For more help welcoming and guiding Spanish-speaking patients, see Chapter 3.

¡Ojo!

The word for bathroom, *el baño*, universally designates public restrooms. However, patients may use regional words when they ask for directions: *el excusado* (excused), *el inodoro* (odorless), *el retrete* (retreat), *el gabinete* (private room), *los servicios* (sanitary services).

Surgery

When the patient needs surgery, too much is at stake to risk misunderstandings. Clear communication is vital now more than ever. The following words and phrases will help you make sure things go smoothly for your Spanish-speaking patients.

First, the names of some common procedures.

Surgical Procedures

appendectomy	apendectomía	ah pehn dehk toh MEE ah
arthroscopy	artroscopía	ahr trohs koh PEE ah
biopsy	biopsia	BYOHP syah
bypass	baipás/derivación	bay PAHS / deh ree vah SYOHN
colostomy	colostomía	koh lohs toh MEE ah

continues

continued

D & C	dilatación y curetaje /raspado	dee lah tah SYOHN ee koo reh TAH heh/ rrahs PAH thoh
hysterectomy	histerectomía	ees teh rehk toh MEE ah
implant	implante	eem PLAHN teh
joint replacement	repuesto de articulación	rreh PWEHS toh theh_ahr tee koo lah SYOHN
mastectomy	mastectomía	mahs tehk toh MEE ah
tonsillectomy	amigdalectomía	ah meeg thah lehk toh MEE ah
tracheostomy	traqueostomía	trah keh ohs toh MEE ah
vasectomy	vasectomía	vah sehk toh MEE ah

Pre-Op Give and Take

Before surgery, patient and staff need to trade vital information. There's high anxiety on the patient's part, a need to know what will happen and why. For their part, the surgical staff needs specific information from the patient, to make sure all goes well. Use the phrases that follow to meet both needs:

This is an operation to …
Esta operación es para …
EHS tah_oh peh rah SYOHN ehs PAH rah …

   drain the infection.
   drenar la infección.
   threh NAHR lah_een fehk SYOHN

fix your heart.
reparar su corazón.
rreh pah RAHR soo koh rah SOHN

improve circulation.
mejorar la circulación.
meh hoh rahr lah seer koo lah SYOHN

relieve the pressure.
reducir la presión.
rreh thoo SEER lah preh SYOHN

remove the tumor.
quitarle el tumor.
kee TAHR leh_ehl too MOHR

remove your ____.
sacarle el/la ____.
sah KAHR leh_ehl/lah ____

repair the damage.
reparar el daño.
rreh pah RAHR ehl THAH nyoh

This operation is (very) …
Esta operación es (muy) …
EHS tah_oh peh rah SYOHN ehs (mooy)

common	común	koh MOON
complicated	complicada	kohm plee KAH thah
dangerous	peligrosa	peh lee GROH sah
necessary	necesaria	neh seh SAH ryah
serious	grave	GRAH veh
simple	sencilla	sehn SEE yah

Have you ever had surgery before?
¿Le han operado antes?
leh_ahn oh peh RAH thoh_AHN tehs

The operation will take ____ hours.
La operación tomará ____ horas.
lah_oh peh rah SYOHN toh mah RAH ____ OH
rahs

We're going to ...
Vamos a ...
BAH mohs ah

> prepare you for the operation.
> prepararle para la operación.
> preh pah RAHR leh PAH rah lah_oh peh rah
> SYOHN

I'm going to give you a sedative now.
Le voy a dar un calmante ahora.
leh voy ah thahr oon kahl MAHN teh_ah OH rah

You will (will not) be awake during the operation.
(No) Estará despierto durante la operación.
(noh_) ehs tah RAH thehs PYEHR toh thoo
RAHN teh lah_oh peh rah SYOHN

I will come out and talk to your family when the
operation is over.
Saldré a hablar con su familia cuando termine la
operación.
sahl THREH_ah_ah VLAHR kohn soo fah MEE
lyah KWAHN doh tehr MEE neh lah_oh peh rah
SYOHN

You will be in the recovery room for ___ hours.
Estará en la sala de recuperación por ___ horas.
ehs tah RAH_ehn lah SAH lah theh rreh koo peh
rah SYOHN pohr ___ OH rahs

When the Operation Is Over

After surgery, the family (and the patient!) will be
anxious to hear the outcome. You'll need the words
to deliver the message, whether it's good news or
bad. The phrases that follow will help:

Through Their Eyes

Show consideration for the patient and
family members in this emotionally
charged moment. See "First, Show That
You Care" in Chapter 7 for appropriate
ways to express your empathy for everyone concerned.

The operation was successful.
La operación fue un éxito.
lah_oh peh rah SYOHN fweh_oon EHK see toh

There are/were complications.
Hay/hubo complicaciones.
AY / OO voh kohm plee kah SYOH nehs

We don't know yet if he (she) will live.
No sabemos si vivirá.
noh sah VEH mohs see vee vee RAH

He (she) died.
Se murió.
seh moo RYOH

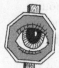

¡Ojo!

You may soften the news of the patient's death without saying "die": He/She couldn't fight any longer: *No pudo resistir más.*

I'm very sorry.
Lo siento muchísimo.
loh SYEHN toh moo CHEE see moh

Nursing Necessities

While patients are in the hospital, nobody interacts with them more than their nurses. Day and night, nurses and nursing assistants are there to guide, explain, comfort, and treat. In the scope of this guide, it's not possible to include all the words an English-speaking nurse might need to care for a Spanish-speaking patient, but here are some of the basics:

The tube is ...
El tubo es ...
ehl TOO voh_ehs

> for IV fluids.
> para líquidos intravenosos.
> PAH rah LEE kee thohs een trah veh NOH sohs
>
> for pain medication.
> para medicamentos para el dolor.
> PAH rah meh thee kah MEHN tohs PAH
> rah_ehl thoh LOHR

to help with breathing.
para ayudarle a respirar.
PAH rah_ah yoo THAHR leh_ah rrehs pee
RAHR

I'm going to …
Voy a …
Boy ah

   change your IV.
   cambiarle la infusión intravenosa.
   kahm BYAHR leh lah_een foo SYOHN een
   trah veh NOH sah

   check …
   averiguar …
   ah veh ree GWAHR

   your temperature.
   su temperatura.
   soo tehm peh rah TOO rah

   your vital signs.
   sus signos vitales.
   soos SEEG nohs vee TAH lehs

   take some blood.
   tomarle un poco de sangre.
   toh MAHR leh_oom POH koh theh SAHN
   greh

Do you need anything for pain?
¿Necesita algo para el dolor?
neh seh SEE tah_ahl goh PAH rah_ehl thoh LOHR

I need to ask the doctor.
Necesito preguntárselo al doctor.
neh seh SEE toh preh goon TAHR seh loh ahl
thohk TOHR

These are the doctor's orders.
Éstas son las órdenes del doctor.
EHS tahs sohn lahs OHR theh nehs thehl thohk
TOHR

The doctor says no.
El médico dice que no.
ehl MEH thee koh thee seh keh noh

You are not well enough yet.
Todavía no está completamente bien.
toh thah VEE ah noh_ehs TAH kkohm pleh tah
MEHN teh vyehn

You need to try to sit up.
Debe tratar de incorporarse.
Deh veh trah TAHR theh_een kohr poh RAHR seh

You need to start walking.
Debe comenzar a caminar.
Deh veh koh mehn SAHR ah kah mee NAHR

Walk slowly.
Camine despacito.
kah MEE neh thehs pah SEE toh

Have you urinated yet?
¿Ya ha orinado?
yah_ah_oh ree NAH thoh

Have you passed gas yet?
¿Ya ha soltado gas?
yah_ah sohl TAH thoh gahs

Visiting Hours

Chances are, your Hispanic patients love having visitors. And visitors are sometimes the best medicine. But hospitals have policies and patients need rest, so when it's time to spell out the restrictions, you'll need these phrases:

Children must be ___ years old to visit patients.
No se admiten niños menores de ___ años para visitar a los pacientes.
noh seh ahth MEE tehn NEE nyohs meh NOH rehs theh ___ AH nyohs PAH rah vee see TAHR ah lohs pah SYEHN tehs

She (he) needs rest now.
Ahora necesita descansar.
ah OH rah neh seh SEE tah thehs kahn SAHR

He (she) isn't seeing any visitors.
No admite ninguna visita.
noh_ahth MEE teh nneen GOO nah vee SEE tah

There are too many visitors in the room.
Hay demasiados visitantes en el cuarto.
ay theh mah SYAH thohs vee see TAHN tehs ehn ehl KWAHR toh

Visiting hours are over.
Las horas de visita ya terminaron.
lahs OH rahs theh vee SEE tah yah tehr mee NAH rohn

When It's Time to Go Home

You've done your job well and the patient is ready to go home. There are just a few things left to cover:

You are being discharged today.
Le van a dar de alta hoy.
leh vahn ah thahr theh_AHL tah_oy

Here are instructions to follow at home.
Aquí tiene las instrucciones que seguir en casa.
ah KEE TYEH neh lahs eens trook SYOH nehs
keh seh GEER ehn KAH sah

Do you have someone to help take care of you
when you are at home?
¿Tiene a alguien que pueda cuidarle cuando vuelva
a su casa?
TYEH neh_ah_AHL gyehn keh PWEH thah
KWEE THAHR leh KWAHN doh VWEHL
vah_ah soo KAH sah

A nurse will come to your home.
Una enfermera irá a su casa.
OO nah_ehn fehr MEH rah_ee RAH_ah soo
KAH sah

This is when you need to see the doctor next.
Esto es cuándo debe ver al médico la próxima vez.
EHS toh_ehs KWAHN doh THEH veh vehr ahl
MEH thee koh lah PROHK see mah vehs

Here are the telephone numbers to call if you have
any problems or questions.
Aquí tiene los números de teléfono para llamarnos
si tiene algún problema o si se le ocurre alguna
pregunta.
ah KEE TYEH neh lohs NOO meh rohs theh teh
LEH foh noh PAH rah yah MAHR nohs see TYEH
neh_ahl GOON proh VLEH mah_oh see seh
leh_oh KOO rreh_ahl GOO nah preh GOON tah

10

Home Health Care Nursing

Medically speaking, providing care in the patient's home may be simply the next step in treatment, but from the patient's perspective, it is much more. Invitation to a Hispanic person's home marks an important milestone in personal relationships, often the promotion from acquaintance (*conocido*) to friend (*amigo*). As a visiting nurse, be aware that you have been admitted into a very special part of the patient's world.

All those in the home are already a part of that intimate circle, so—each time you come—acknowledge their importance by taking a moment to greet all those present, even if they have not been formally introduced to you. A cordial *¡Buenos días! ¿Cómo está?* (Hello! How are you?) will assure you of everyone's collaboration in caring for the patient.

And one other thing: Hispanics consider it impolite to notice and comment on the home or its contents. What to an English speaker are innocent compliments about the house and its furnishings will have your hosts talking about you after you've left. Of course, if you see something that poses a hazard or impacts the patient's care, you'll need to speak up. But steer clear of the décor when exchanging pleasantries.

The First Visit

When you first see a patient in his or her home, you'll want to introduce yourself, explain why and when you'll be visiting, and assess certain basics about the patient's condition and environment. Use the following phrases to lay the groundwork.

I am your visiting nurse.
Soy la enfermera (el enfermero) de visita.
soy lah_ehn fehr MEH rah (ehl_ehn fehr MEH roh) theh vee SEE tah

My name is _____.
Me llamo _____.
meh YAH moh

Your doctor wants me to see you until you are a bit better.
Su médico desea que le vea hasta que se sienta un poco mejor.
soo MEH thee koh theh SEH ah keh leh VEH ah_AHS tah keh seh SYEHN tah_oom POH koh meh HOHR

Do you live alone?
¿Vive solo? (sola)
BEE veh SOH loh (SOH lah)

Who lives with you here?
¿Con quién vive usted?
kohn kyehm BEE veh_oos TEHTH

Are they able and willing to help you?
¿Están dispuestos (dispuestas) y listos (listas) para
ayudarle?
ehs TAHN thees PWEHS tohs (thees PWEHS
tahs) ee LEES tohs (LEES tahs) PAH rah ah yoo
THAHR leh

Is a friend or neighbor able and willing to help you?
¿Tiene un amigo o vecino dispuesto y capaz de
ayudarle?
TYEH neh_oon ah MEE goh_oh veh SEE noh
thees PWEHS toh_ee kah PAHS theh_ah yoo
THAHR leh

I need to meet him/her to talk about your medical
needs.
Necesito conocerlo (conocerla) para hablarle de sus
necesidades médicas.
neh seh SEE toh koh noh SEHR loh (koh noh
SEHR lah) PAH rah_ah VLAHR leh theh soos neh
seh see THAH thehs MEH thee kahs

I need to do a safety check of your home.
Necesito revisar su casa para asegurarme de que
nada le ponga a riesgo.
neh seh SEE toh rreh vee SAHR soo KAH sah
PAH rah_ah seh goo RAHR meh theh keh NAH
thah leh POHN gah_ah RYEHS goh

Can you do your own personal hygiene?
¿Puede hacer su aseo personal sin ayuda?
PWEH theh_ah SEHR soo_ah SEH oh pehr soh
NAHL seen ah YOO thah

Can you dress (undress) yourself?
¿Puede ponerse (quitarse) la ropa sin ayuda?
PWEH theh poh NEHR seh (kee TAHR seh) lah
RROH pah seen ah YOO thah

Can you prepare meals by yourself?
¿Puede prepararse la comida sin ayuda?
PWEH theh preh pah RAHR seh lah koh MEE
thah seen ah YOO thah

Can you walk without assistance?
¿Puede caminar sin ayuda?
PWEH theh kah mee NAHR seen ah YOO thah

Can you get in and out of your chair by yourself?
¿Puede sentarse y levantarse de la silla sin ayuda?
PWEH theh sehn TAHR she_ee leh vahn TAHR
she then lah SEE yah seen ah YOO thah

Let me see you …
Permítame verle …
pehr MEE tah meh vehr leh

> get out of bed.
> levantarse de la cama.
> leh vahn TAHR seh theh lah KAH mah

> walk.
> caminar.
> kah mee NAHR

> use the telephone.
> usar el teléfono.
> oo SAHR ehl teh LEH foh noh

Please read these instructions to me.
A ver, léame estas instrucciones.
ah vehr, LEH ah meh_EHS tahs eens trook SYOH
nehs

Do you have memory problems?
¿Tiene problema con la memoria?
TYEH neh proh VLEH mah kohn lah meh MOH
ryah

I am ordering some medical equipment for you.
Voy a pedir equipo médico para su uso.
boy ah peh THEER eh KEE poh MEH thee koh
PAH rah soo_OO soh

[Insert from below] will see you soon.
[…] vendrá a verle pronto.
vehn DRAH_ah VEHR leh PROHN toh

> A physical therapist …
> Un terapeuta …
> oon teh rah PEW tah

> A home health aide for your bath (meals) …
> Un asistente casero (una asistenta casera)
> para sus baños (comidas) …
> oon ah sees TEHN teh kah SEH roh (OO
> nah_ah sees TEHN tah kah SEH rah) PAH
> rah soos BAH nyohs (koh MEE thahs)

> A social worker …
> Un trabajador social …
> oon trah vah hah THOHR soh SYAHL

I am going to set up a meal delivery service for you.
Voy a empezarle el servicio de entrega de comidas
preparadas.

boy ah_ehm peh SAHR leh_ehl sehr VEE syoh
theh_ehn TREH gah theh koh MEE thahs preh
pah RAH thahs

The doctor wants to see you again on _____.
El médico desea verle de nuevo el _____.
ehl MEH thee koh theh SEH ah VEHR leh theh
NWEH voh_ehl

I will see you again on _____ at _____ A.M. (P.M.).
Volveré a verle el _____ a la(s) _____ de la mañana
(tarde).
bohl veh REH_ah VEHR leh_ehl _____ ah lah(s) _____
theh lah mah NYAH nah (TAHR theh)

Medication

A big part of home care is making sure patients are
taking their medications properly. First, you'll want
to see that they've disposed of their old medications:

Where are (Let me see) your old medications?
¿Dónde tiene (Permítame ver) sus viejas medicinas?
Dohn deh TYEH neh (pehr MEE tah meh vehr)
soos VYEH hahs meh thee SEE nahs

Let's get rid of these now.
Botemos estos ahora.
boh TEH mohs EHS tohs ah OH rah

After the old medications are gone, you can sort
out what they *should* be taking:

Let's go over your new medicines.
Repasemos sus nuevas medicinas.
rreh pah SEH mohs soos NWEH vahs meh thee
SEE nahs

Tell me what you understand about them.
Acláreme lo que usted comprende sobre ellas.
ah KLAH reh meh loh keh_oos TEHTH kohm
PREHN deh SOH vreh_EH yahs

Who gives you your medications?
¿Quién le da sus medicinas?
kyehn leh thah soos meh thee SEE nahs

I will put your medications in a weekly/daily con-
tainer so you won't make any mistakes.
Pondré sus medicamentos en un dosificador
semanal /diario para evitar errores.
pohn DREH soos meh thee kah MEHN tohs ehn
oon doh see fee kah thohr seh man NAHL /DYAH
ryoh /PAH rah_eh vee TAHR eh RROH rehs

I will leave you a chart of medication instructions.
Le daré una hoja de instrucciones para sus medicamentos.
leh thah REH_OO nah_OH hah theh_eens trook
SYOH nehs PAH rah soos meh thee kah MEHN
tohs

Wound Care

If the patient has a new incision or other wound,
you'll want to be sure he or she knows how to care
for it:

Can you change your own bandage?
¿Puede usted cambiarse la venda?
PWEH theh_oos TEHTH kahm BYAHR seh lah
VEHN dah

Show me how you do it.
Permítame ver cómo lo hace.
pehr MEE tah meh vehr KOH moh loh AH seh

Watch me, I will show you what to do.
Míreme, le mostraré cómo se hace.
MEE reh meh, leh mohs trah REH KOH moh seh
AH seh

Do you have any questions about how to do this?
¿Le queda alguna duda de cómo se hace?
leh KEH thah_ahl GOO nah THOO thah theh
KOH moh seh AH seh

You need to watch for infection.
Vigile bien que no se infecte esto.
bee HEE leh vyehn keh noh seh_een FEHK
teh_EHS toh

Whenever possible, keep it elevated.
Cuando pueda, eleve.
KWAHN doh PWEH thah, eh LEH veh

For more wound care phrases, and instructions about infection, see Chapter 8.

For Catheter Cases

Catheters create risks and demand ongoing management.

Your catheter makes you susceptible to urinary infections.
El catéter le pone a mas riesgo de infecciones urinarias.
ehl kah TEH tehr leh POH neh_ah mahs RYEHS
goh theh_een fehk SYOH nehs oo ree NAH ryahs

Therefore you must …
Por eso usted debe …
pohr EH soh oos TEHTH theh veh

> drink lots of fluids, including cranberry juice,
> every day.
> tomar mucho líquido todos los días, incluso
> jugo dearándano.
> toh MAHR MOO choh LEE kee thoh TOH
> thohs lohs THEE ahs, een KLOO soh HOO
> goh theh_ah RAHN dah noh
>
> keep the tube below your bladder so urine does
> not flow backward.
> procurar que el tubo quede más bajo que la
> vejiga para que la orina no refluya hacia la vejiga.
> proh koo rahr keh_ehl TOO voh KEH theh
> mahs BAH hoh keh lah veh HEE gah PAH rah
> keh lah_oh REE nah no rreh FLOO yah_AH
> syah lah veh HEE gah

If you see blood or pus in the bag or tube, call the
agency or doctor.
Si nota que hay sangre o pus en la bolsa o el tubo,
llame al médico o a la agencia.
see NOH tah keh_ay SAHN greh_oh poos ehn lah
BOHL sah_oh_ehl TOO voh, YAH meh_ahl MEH
thee koh_oh_ah lah_ah HEHN syah

If it stops flowing, check for kinks or objects
obstructing the flow.
Si la corriente de orina se interrumpe, busque la
torcedura u otra obstucción responsable.

see lah koh RRYEHN teh theh_oh REE nah
seh_een teh RROOM peh, BOOS keh lah tohr seh
THOO rah_oo_OH trah_ohvs trook SYOHN
rrehs pohn SAH vleh

If urine is still not flowing and you are beginning
to feel pressure, call the agency, day or night.
Si la orina todavía no fluye y usted comienza a
sentir presión, llame a la agencia a cualquier hora,
día y noche.
see lah_oh REE nah toh thah VEE ah noh FLOO
yeh_ee_oos TEHTH koh MYEHN sah_ah sehn
TEER preh SYOHN, YAH meh_ah lah_ah
HEHN syah_ah kwahl KYEHR OH rah, THEE
ah_ee NOH cheh

If you have a fever higher than 100 degrees, call
the agency or your doctor.
Si tiene una fiebre de más de cien grados, llame al
médico o a la agencia.
see TYEH neh_OO nah FYEH vreh theh mahs
theh syehn GRAH thohs, YAH meh_ahl MEH
thee koh_oh_ah lah_ah HEHN syah

I am going to leave extra catheters here for future
use.
Voy a dejarle catéteres extras para usar en el futuro.
boy ah theh HAHR leh kah TEH teh rehs EHS
trahs PAH rah_oo SAHR ehn ehl foo TOO roh

Through Their Eyes

Recent immigrants are accustomed to the Celsius scale, not the Fahrenheit scale. To be sure they understand your instructions, remember to give temperatures in Celsius as well as Fahrenheit.

For Diabetic Cases

A diagnosis of diabetes can bring some abrupt lifestyle changes and demanding medication regimens. It's not an easy condition to manage.

Do you know how to test your blood sugar?
¿Sabe hacer la prueba de glucosa en la sangre?
SAH veh_ah SEHR lah PRWEH vah theh gloo KOH sah_ehn lah SAHN greh

Show me how you do it.
Muéstreme cómo la hace.
MWEHS treh meh KOH moh lah_AH seh

You must test your blood sugar as the doctor prescribed.
Debe hacer la prueba de glucosa como se la indicó el médico.
DEH veh_ah SEHR lah PRWEH vah theh gloo KOH moh seh lah_een dee KOH_ehl MEH thee koh

Show me how you prepare and give your insulin shot.
Muéstreme cómo prepara la inyección de insulina y cómo se la pone.
MWEHS treh meh KOH mo preh PAH rah lah_een yehk SYOHN deh_een soo LEE nah_ee KOH moh seh lah POH neh

I will prepare your insulin for you.
Le prepararé la insulina.
leh preh pah rah REH lah_een soo LEE nah

You can keep several doses in the refrigerator, along with the insulin vials.
Puede guardar varias dosificaciones en la refrigeradora, con los frascos de insulina.
PWEH theh gwahr THAHR VAH ryahs thoh see fee kah SYOH nehs ehn lah rreh free heh rah THOH rah kohn lohs FRAHS kohs theh_een soo LEE nah

For more help in discussing diabetes care with patients, see Chapter 8.

For Postpartum

A new life in the family means joy; it also means special needs and a period of adjustment.

I have to check on you and the baby.
Tengo que averiguar cómo están usted y el bebé.
TEHN goh keh_ah veh ree GWAHR KOH moh_ehs TAHN oos TEHTH ee_ehl veh VEH

Is the baby eating well?
¿Come bien el bebé?
KOH meh vyehn ehl veh VEH

Are there problems?
¿Hay algún problema?
ay ahl GOOM proh VLEH mah

Has the baby had a bowel movement yet?
¿Ya ha defecado el bebé?
yah_ah theh feh KAH thoh_ehl veh VEH

Did you see blood?
¿Notó si había sangre?
noh TOH see_ah VEE_ah SAHN greh

I have to do a blood test from the baby's foot.
Tengo que sacarle al bebé una muestra de la sangre
del pie.
TEHN goh keh sah KAHR leh_ahl veh VEH_OO
nah MWEHS trah theh lah SAHN greh thehl pyeh

If this test is normal, you will *not* hear from us
about it.
No le avisaremos del resultado a menos que sean
anormales.
noh leh ah vee sah REH mohs thehl rreh sool TAH
thoh_ah MEH nohs keh SEH ahn ah nohr MAH lehs

How are you doing?
¿Cómo le va?
KOH moh leh vah

I need to check your Caesarean-section incision.
Necesito revisarle la incisión cesárea.
neh seh SEE toh reh vee SAHR leh lah_een see
SYOHN seh SAH reh ah

I need to change the bandage.
Tengo que cambiarle la venda.
TEHN goh keh kahm BYAHR leh lah VEHN dah

For now you may only shower.
Por ahora sólo puede ducharse.
pohr ah OH rah SOH loh PWEH theh thoo
CHAHR seh

Take your temperature every four hours for ___ more days.

Tómese la temperatura cada cuatro horas por ___ días más.

TOH meh seh lah tehm peh rah TOO rah KAH thah KWAH troh_OH rahs pohr ___ THEE ahs mahs

Call the agency or the doctor if you or the baby has a fever.

Llame a la agencia o al médico si usted o el bebé tiene fiebre.

YAH meh_ah lah_ah HEHN syah_oh_ahl MEH thee koh see_oos TEHTH oh_ehl veh VEH TYEH neh FYEH vreh

You should wait six weeks to have intercourse.

No debe tener relaciones sexuales por seis semanas.

noh THEH veh teh NEHR rreh lah SYOH nehs sehk SWAH lehs pohr seys MEH sehs

Are you breastfeeding?

¿Le da el pecho?

leh thah_ehl PEH choh

Are you having any problems with breastfeeding?

¿Tiene algún problema al dárselo?

TYEH neh_ahl GOOM proh VLEH mah_ahl DAHR seh loh

Breastfeeding is *not* effective birth control; you can still get pregnant.

No es cierto que el dar el pecho sea contraceptivo; siempre puede concebir.

noh_ehs SYEHR toh keh_ehl thahr ehl PEH choh SEH ah kohn trah sehp TEE voh; SYEHM preh PWEH theh kohn seh VEER

For Respiratory Cases

Patients who have trouble breathing often have some new equipment in their lives.

I am going to have oxygen delivered today.
Voy a ordenar que entreguen su oxígeno hoy.
boy ah_ohr theh NAHR keh_ehn TREH gehn
soo_ohk SEE heh noh_oy

Do you know how to use your inhaler?
¿Sabe usar su inhalador?
SAh veh_oo SAHR soo_een ah lah THOHR

Let me show you the proper way.
Permítame mostrarle el modo apropiado.
pehr MEE tah meh mohs TRAHR leh_ehl MOH
thoh_ah proh PYAH thoh

To use your inhaler:
Para usar su inhalador:
PAH rah_oo SAHR soo_een ah lah THOHR

> Shake it.
> Agítelo.
> ah HEE teh loh
>
> Inhale one puff.
> Aspire una atomización.
> ahs PEE reh_OO nah_ah toh mee sah SYOHN
>
> Hold your breath for as long as possible.
> Aguante el aliento lo más posible.
> ah GWAHN teh_ehl ah LYEHN toh loh mahs
> poh SEE vleh

Wait 30 to 60 seconds.
Espere desde treinta a sesenta segundos.
ehs PEH reh THEHS theh TREYN tah_ah
seh SEHN tah seh GOON dohs

Then inhale the second puff …
Luego aspire la segunda atomización …
LWEH goh_ahs PEE reh lah seh GOON dah_ah
toh mee sah SYOHN

   … and hold it as long as possible.
   … y aguántela lo más posible.
   … ee ah GWAHN teh lah loh mahs poh SEE
   vleh

11

OB/GYN

In the Hispanic culture, the roles of men and women are clearly defined, and though times change, 2,000 years of culture is hard to shake off, especially in poor rural areas. Certain things are considered the business of men, and others are women's territory. Firmly in the latter are women's health and reproductive issues.

Traditionally, Hispanic women have helped and cared for each other through the experiences of womanhood—older women guiding younger through puberty, pregnancy, childbirth, and menopause. If you're a woman practicing OB/GYN, your Hispanic patients will find it natural to confide in you. But if you're a man, you'll need to be especially sensitive to their ingrained reluctance to let you treat them, or even to discuss these personal matters with you.

Words for Women's Health

English	Spanish	Pronunciation
amniotic sac	la bolsa amniótica	lah BOHL sah_ah NYOH tee kah
anus	el ano	ehl AH noh
breasts	los senos	lohs SEH nohs
birth canal	el canal cervical	ehl kah NAHL sehr vee KAHL
cervix	el cuello uterino	ehl KWEH yoh_oo teh REE noh
embryo	el embrión	ehl ehm BRYOHN
erection	la erección	lah_eh rehk SYOHN
fallopian tubes	las trompas de falopio	lahs TROHM pahs theh fah LOH pyoh
fertilization	la fertilización	lah fehr tee lee sah SYOHN
fetus	el feto	ehl FEH toh
genes	los genes	lohs HEH nehs
hormones	las hormonas	lahs ohr MOH nahs
intercourse	el coito	ehl KOY toh
menopause	la menopausia	lah meh noh POW syah
menstrual cycle	el ciclo menstrual	ehl SEE kloh mehns TRWAHL
menstrual period	la menstruación (medical)	lah mehns trwah SYOHN
	la regla (popular)	lah RREH glah
navel	el ombligo	ehl ohm BLEE goh
nipple	el pezón	ehl peh SOHN
obstetrician	el obstetra	ehl ovs TEH trah

ovary	el ovario	ehl oh VAH ryoh
ovum	el óvulo	ehl OH voo loh
penis	el pene	ehl PEH neh
placenta	la placenta	lah plah SEHN tah
pubic hair	el vello púbico	ehl VEH yoh POO bee koh
scrotum	el escroto	ehl ehs KROH toh
semen	el semen	ehl SEH mehn
sperm	la esperma	lah ehs PER mah
testicles	los testículos	lohs tehs TEE koo lohs
umbilical cord	el cordón umbilical	ehl kohr THOHN oom bee lee KAHL
urethra	la uretra	lah_oo REH trah
vagina	la vagina	lah vah HEE nah
vulva	la vulva	lah VOOL vah

The Healthy Woman

During any gynecological exam, you'll need certain information. The phrases in this section will help you gather it.

History

Note: For ways to ask about the patient's general medical history, see Chapter 4. For more questions to help you examine the patient, see Chapter 5.

Menstrual Cycle

When was your last period?
¿Cuándo fue su última regla?
KWAHN doh fweh soo_OOL tee mah RREH glah

How old were you when you had your first menstrual cycle (period)?
¿Cuántos años tenía cuando tuvo su primera regla?
KWAHN tohs AH nyohs teh NEE ah KWAHN doh TOO voh soo pree MEH rah RREH glah

Do you still have it now?
¿Sigue teniéndola todavía?
SEE geh teh NYEHN doh lah toh thah VEE ah

How many days pass between periods?
¿A cada cuántos días le viene la regla?
ah KAH thah KWAHN tohs THEE ahs leh VYEH neh lah RREH glah

Do you bleed between your periods?
¿Le sale sangre en el intervalo entre reglas?
leh SAH leh SAHN greh_ehn ehl een tehr VAH loh_ehn treh RREH glahs

| a little? | un poco | oom POH koh |
| a lot? | mucho | MOO choh |

Breast Health

When was your last …
¿Cuándo fue su último …
KWAHN doh fweh soo_OOL tee mo

breast examination?
examen del seno?
ehk SAH mehn thehl SEH noh

mammogram?
mamograma?
mah moh GRAH mah

Were the results normal?
¿Dio resultado normal?
dyoh rreh sool TAH thoh nohr MAHL

Have you noticed any …
¿Ha notado cualquier …
ah noh TAH thoh kwahl KYEHRA

  change in …
  cambio en …
  KAHM byoh_ehn

      your breasts?
      el tamaño de los senos?
      ehl tah MAH nyoh theh lohs
      SEH nohs

      your nipples?
      los pezones?
      lohs peh SOH nehs

      under your arms?
      debajo de los brazos?
      theh VAH hoh theh lohs
      BRAH sohs

Do you know how to examine your breasts?
¿Sabe examinarse los senos?
SAH veh_ehk sah mee NAHR seh lohs SEH nohs

I will show you how.
Le mostraré cómo se hace.
leh mohs trah REH KOH moh seh_AH seh

It is important that you examine your breasts regularly.
Es importante que se examine los senos regularmente.
ehs eem pohr TAHN teh keh seh_ehk sah MEE neh
lohs SEH nos rreh goo lahr MEHN teh

The best time to examine your breasts is after your
period.
El momento más oportuno para examinarse los
senos es después de la regla.
ehl moh MEHN toh mahs oh pohr TOO noh PAH
rah_ehk sah mee NAHR seh lohs SEH nohs ehs
thehs PWEHS theh lah RREH glah

Past Pregnancies

Do you have any hereditary diseases?
¿Tiene usted alguna enfermedad hereditaria?
TYEH neh_oos TEHTH ahl GOO nah_ehn fehr
meh THAHTH eh reh thee TAH ryah

How many pregnancies and live births have you had?
¿Cuántas veces ha tenido embarazos y partos vivos?
KWAHN tahs VEH sehs ah teh NEE thoh_ehm
bah RAH sohs ee PAHR tohs VEE vohs

Were all your pregnancies normal?
¿Fueron todos sus embarazos normales?
FWEH rohn TOH thohs soos ehm bah RAH sohs
nohr MAH lehs

Have you had …
¿Ha tenido …
ah teh NEE thoh

> multiple births?
> partos múltiples?
> PAHR tohs MOOL tee plehs

twins?
gemelos?
heh MEH lohs

more than two?
más de dos?
mahs theh thohs

a child that was born ...
un bebé que salió ...
oon veh VEH keh sah LYOH

> feet first?
> los pies primero?
> lohs pyehs pree MEH roh
>
> with the cord wrapped around
> his/her neck?
> con el cordón enroscado al cuello?
> kohn ehl kohr THOHN ehn
> rohs KAH thoh_ahl KWEH yoh
>
> and died shortly after birth?
> y luego murió poco después de
> nacer?
> ee LWEH goh moo RYOH
> POH koh thehs PWEHS theh
> nah SEHR
>
> dead?
> muerto?
> MWEHR toh

a forceps delivery?
un parto con fórceps?
oon PAHR toh kohn FOHR sehps

a Caesarean delivery?
una cesárea?
OO nah seh SAH reh ah

problems with the placenta?
algún problema con la placenta?
ahl GOOM proh VLEH mah kohn lah plah
SEHN tah

a postpartum hemorrhage?
una hemorragia después del parto?
OO nah_eh moh RRAH hyah thehs PWEHS
thehl PAHR toh

a miscarriage?
un aborto espontáneo?
oon ah VOHR toh ehs pohn TAH neh oh

Physical Exam and Pap Smear

Are you bleeding?
¿Está sangrando ahora?
ehs TAH sahn GRAHN doh_ah OH rah

I am going to examine …
Le voy a examinar …
leh voy ah_ehk sah mee NAHR

your breasts.	los senos.	lohs SEH nohs
your genitals.	los genitales.	lohs heh nee TAH lehs
your pelvis.	el pelvis.	ehl PEHL vees

Please ...
Por favor ...
pohr fah VOHR

> remove your underwear.
> quítese la ropa interior.
> KEE teh seh lah RROH pah_een teh RYOHR

> bear down.
> puje.
> POO heh

> slide closer to the end of the table.
> córrase más cerca del borde de la mesa.
> KOH rrah seh mahs SEHR kah thehl VOHR
> theh theh lah MEH sah

> put your legs up here.
> ponga las piernas aquí.
> POHN gah lahs PYEHR nahs ah KEE

Are you breastfeeding now?
¿Está dando el pecho ahora?
ehs TAH THAHN doh ehl PEH choh_ah OH rah

Do you have herpes?
¿Tiene herpe(s)?
TYEH neh_EHR peh(s)

Contraception

The following table lists words for the primary
forms of contraception. After the table, you'll find
phrases to help make sure your patients know how
to use them effectively.

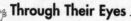

Through Their Eyes

With your Hispanic patients, it may be best to address contraception as a health issue rather than a way to avoid bearing (more) children. For many Hispanic women, particularly those of humble origin who obey God, their priest, their husband, and their father (in that order), pregnancy is what is supposed to happen.

Forms of Contraception

abstinence	abstinencia	ahvs tee NEHN syah
birth control pills	las píldoras anticonceptivas	lahs PEEL thoh rahs ahn tee kohn sehp TEE vahs
coitus interruptus	la interrupción de coito	lah_een teh rroop SYOHN theh KOY toh
condoms	los condones	lohs kohn DOH nehs
creams	las cremas	lahs KREH mahs
diaphragm	el diafragma	ehl dyah FRAHG mah
foams	las espumas	lahs ehs POO mahs
IUD	el aparato intrauterino	ehl ah pah RAH toh_een trow teh REE noh
rhythm method	el método de ritmo	ehl MEH toh thoh theh RREET moh

| tubal ligation | la ligadura de los tubos | lah lee gah THOO rah theh lohs TOO vohs |
| vasectomy | la vasectomía | lah vah sehk toh MEE ah |

Note: Many women, and not just Latinas, think that if they are breastfeeding, they can't get pregnant. That's a myth, and it's important you debunk it. Say:

Breastfeeding is *not* effective birth control; you can still get pregnant while nursing a baby.
El dar el pecho no es de ninguna manera contraceptivo; siempre puede concebir.
ehl thahr ehl PEH choh noh_ehs theh neen GOO nah mah NEH rah kohn trah sehp TEE voh, SYEHM preh PWEH theh kohn seh VEER

Taking the Birth Control Pill

You must follow all the instructions for it to be effective.
Tiene que seguir todas las instrucciones para que la píldora le proteja debidamente.
TYEH neh keh seh GEER TOH thahs lahs eens trook SYOH nehs PAH rah keh lah PEEL thoh rah leh proh TEH hah theh vee thah MEHN teh

Using a Condom and Foam

You must use the foam and a condom at the same time.
Use la espuma y un condón al mismo tiempo.
OO seh lah_ehs POO mah_ee_oon kohn DOHN ahl MEES moh TYEHM poh

Use the foam no more than ___ hours before intercourse.

Use la espuma no más de ____ horas antes del acto sexual.

OO seh lah_ehs POO mah noh mahs theh ___ OH rahs AHN tehs thehl AHK toh sehk SWAHL

The man should wear the condom during the entire sexual episode.

El hombre debe usar el condón toda la duración de relaciones íntimas.

ehl OHM breh THEH veh_oo SAHR ehl kohn DOHN TOH thah lah thoo rah SYOHN theh lahs rreh lah SYOH nehs EEN tee mahs

Condoms do not always protect against sexually transmitted disease.

Los condones no deben considerarse como protección contra las enfermedades trasmitidas sexualmente.

lohs kohn DOH nehs noh THEH vehn kohn see theh RAHR seh KOH moh proh tehk SYOHN KOHN trah lahs ehn fehr meh THAH thehs trahs mee TEE thahs sehk swahl MEHN teh

Avoid douching unless a medical professional tells you to.

Evite el lavado vaginal a menos que se lo indique un practicante médico.

eh VEE teh_ehl lah VAH thoh vah hee NAHL ah MEH nohs keh seh loh_een DEE keh_oom prahk tee KAHN teh MEH thee koh

Using a Diaphragm

Put the diaphragm in place _____ hours before having intercourse.

Emplace el diafragma _____ horas antes de tener relaciones sexuales.

ehm PLAH seh_ehl thyah FRAHG mah ___ OH rahs AHN tehs theh teh NEHR rreh lah SYOH nehs sehk SWAH lehs

Put the special cream on the diaphragm before putting it in.

Aplique la crema especial al diafragma antes de insertárselo.

ah PLEE keh lah KREH mah ehs peh SYAHL_ahl thyah FRAHG mah AHN tehs theh_een sehr TAHR seh loh

Remove the diaphragm _____ hours after intercourse.

Quítese el diafragma ___ horas después del coito.

KEE teh seh_ehl thyah FRAHG mah ___ OH rahs thehs PWEHS thehl KOY toh

Using an IUD

If you wish to use an IUD, I will place it for you.

Si desea usar un aparato intrauterino, yo se lo puedo emplazar.

see theh SEH ah_oo SAHR oon ah pah RAH toh_een trau teh REE noh, yoh seh loh PWEH thoh_ehm plah SAHR

In its proper place, the string will always be the same length.

En su sitio debido, la cuerda siempre tendrá el mismo largo.

ehn soo SEE tyoh theh VEE thoh, lah KWEHR thah SYEHM preh tehn DRAH_ehl MEES moh LAHR goh

You can check the length by inserting your finger.

Compruébelo introduciendo el dedo.

kohm PRWEH veh loh_een troh thoo SYEHN doh_ehl THEH thoh

You can leave the IUD in place for ____ before it needs to be removed.

Puede dejar emplazado el aparato intrauterino por ____ antes de que sea necesario sacarlo.

PWEH theh theh HAHR ehm plah SAH thoh ehl ah pah RAH toh_een trow teh REE noh pohr ____ AHN tehs the que SEH ah neh seh SAH ryoh sah KAHR loh

Only a medical professional should remove the IUD.

Sólo un practicante médico debe sacarle el aparato.

SOH loh_oom prahk tee KAHN teh MEH thee koh THEH veh sah KAHR leh_ehl ah pah RAH toh

Using the Rhythm Method

This method works best if you have very regular periods.

Este método conviene si tiene la regla muy puntual.

EHS teh MEH toh thoh kohn VYEH neh see TYEH neh lah RREH glah muy poon TWAHL

Intercourse from day one of your period to day _____,
then from about day _____ until your period starts
again, usually does not result in pregnancy.

El coito desde el primer día de su regla hasta el día
_____, luego desde el día _____ hasta que vuelva a
tener la próxima regla, generalmente no resulta en
embarazo.

ehl KOY toh THEHS theh_ehl pree MEHR THEE
ah theh soo RREH glah AHS tah_ehl THEE ah
_____, LWEH goh THEHS theh ehl THEE ah _____
AHS tah keh VWEHL vah_ah teh NEHR lah
PROHK see mah RREH glah heh neh rahl MEHN
teh noh rreh SOOL tah_ehn ehm bah RRAH soh

Avoid intercourse at any other time if you use no
other type of contraception.

Evite las relaciones sexuales en otras ocasiones si no
se sirve simultáneamente de otro modo contraceptivo.

eh VEE lahs rreh lah SYOH nehs sehk SWAH lehs
ehn OH trahs oh kah SYOH nehs see noh seh SEER
veh see mool tah neh ah MEHN teh theh_OH troh
MOH thoh kohn trah sehp TEE voh

Sperm can live in your tubes 48 hours after intercourse.

La esperma puede vivir en sus trompas hasta
cuarenta y ocho horas después del coito.

lah_ehs PEHR mah PWEH theh vee VEER ehn
soos TROHM pahs AHS tah kwah REHN tay OH
choh OH rahs thehs PWEHS thehl KOY toh

If you ovulate during that time, you can get pregnant.

Si suelta un óvulo durante ese período, puede concebir.

see SWEHL tah oon OH voo loh thoo RAHN
teh_EH seh peh REE oh thoh, PWEH theh kohn
seh VEER

Pregnancy

Pregnancy has a vocabulary all its own. Here are some terms and phrases you'll need to use with your pregnant patient:

abortion	el aborto (provocado)	ehl ah VOHR toh (proh voh KAH thoh)
adoption	la adopción	lah_ah thohp SYOHN
amniocentesis	el amniocentesis	ehl ahm nyoh sehn TEH sees
breastfeeding (mother)	el dar el pecho	ehl thahr ehl PEH choh
breastfeeding (infant)	el mamar	ehl mah MAHR
contractions	las contracciones	lahs kohn trahk SYOH nehs
diet	la dieta	lah THYEH tah
drug use	el uso de drogas	ehl OO soh theh THROH gahs
exercise	el ejercicio	ehl eh hehr SEE syoh
family planning	la planificación familiar	la plah nee fee kah SYOHN fah mee LYAHR
gestational diabetes	la diabetes debido al embarazo	lah thyah VEH tehs theh VEE thoh_ahl ehm bah RAH soh
labor	el parto	ehl PAHR toh
Lamaze method	el método de Lamaze	ehl MEH toh thoh theh lah MAHS
natural childbirth	el parto natural	ehl PAHR toh nah too RAHL

postpartum depression	la depresión después del parto	lah theh preh SYOHN thehs PWEHS thehl PAHR toh
prenatal care	la atención prenatal	lah_ah tehn SYOHN preh nah TAHL
sonogram	el sonograma	ehl soh noh GRAH mah
sexual relations	las relaciones sexuales	lahs rreh lah SYOH nehs sehk SWAH lehs
stress	el estrés / la tensión emocional	ehl ehs TREHS / lah tehn SYOHN eh moh syoh NAHL
swollen ankles	los tobillos hinchados	lohs toh VEE yohs een CHAH thohs
ultrasound	el ultrasonido	ehl ool trah soh NEE thoh

You are ___ weeks pregnant.
Usted tiene ___ semanas de embarazo.
oos TEHTH TYEH neh ___ seh MAH nahs theh_ehm bah RAH soh

Do you want to …
¿Quiere …
KYEH reh

continue with the pregnancy?
seguir con el embarazo?
seh GEER kohn ehl ehm bah RAH soh

(have) an abortion?
un aborto provocado?
oon ah VOHR toh proh voh KAH thoh

You should not gain more than ____ pounds. ____
(kilograms)
No debe ganar más de ____ libras. (____ kilos)
noh THEH veh gah NAHR mahs theh ___ LEE
vrahs (___ KEE lohs)

For the sake of yourself and your baby, you must
not ...
Por el bienestar de usted y el de su bebé, usted no
debe ...
pohr ehl vyehn ehs TAHR theh_oos TEHTH
ee_ehl theh soo veh VEH, oos TEHTH noh
THEH veh ...

> smoke.
> fumar.
> foo MAHR
> drink alcohol.
> tomar bebidas alcohólicas.
> toh MAHR veh VEE thahs ahl koh OH lee
> kahs
> take any drugs or medications not prescribed
> by your doctor.
> tomar drogas o medicamentos que no hayan
> sido recetados por su doctor.
> toh MAHR THROH gahs oh meh thee kah
> MEHN tohs keh noh_AH yahn SEE thoh rreh
> seh TAH thohs pohr soo thohk TOHR

It is important that you take good care of yourself:
Es importante que usted se cuide mucho:
ehs eem pohr TAHN teh keh_oos TEHTH seh
KWEE theh MOO choh

Eat properly.
Coma prudentemente.
KOH mah proo THEHN teh MEHN teh

Get proper, approved exercise.
Haga ejercicios apropiados aprobados.
AH gah_eh hehr SEE syohs ah proh PYAH
thohs ah proh VAH thohs

Get plenty of rest.
Descanse mucho.
dehs KAHN seh MOO choh

Take these prenatal vitamins.
Tome estas vitaminas prenatales.
TOH meh_EHS tahs vee tah MEE nahs preh
nah TAH lehs

Labor

You are having contractions.
Tiene contracciones.
TYEH neh kohn trahk SYOH nehs

Your water has broken.
Tiene la fuente.
TYEH neh lah FWEHN teh

How close together are the pains?
¿A cada cuánto le vienen los dolores?
ah KAH thah KWAHN toh leh VYEH nehn lohs
thoh LOH rehs

How long does each pain last?
¿Cuánto dura cada dolor?
KWAHN toh THOO rah KAH thah thoh LOHR

You are ___ centimeters dilated.
Tiene ___ centímetros de cuello.
TYEH neh ___ sehn TEE meh trohs theh KWEH yoh

Tell me when you have a pain.
Avíseme cuando tenga un dolor.
ah VEE seh meh KWAHN doh TEHN gah_oon doh
LOHR

Relax your muscles.
Relájese los músculos.
rreh LAH heh seh lohs MOOS koo lohs

Breathe slowly through your mouth.
Respire lentamente por la boca.
rrehs PEE reh lehn tah MEHN teh pohr lah VOH kah

Pant.
Jadee.
hah THEH eh

Don't push yet.
No puje todavía.
noh POO heh toh thah VEE ah

Conserve your strength.
Conserve sus fuerzas.
kohn SEHR veh soos FWEHR sahs

Rest between pains.
Descanse entre los dolores.
dehs KAHN seh_ehn treh lohs thoh LOH rehs

Delivery

Here are words and phrases you'll need during the
delivery itself:

pull	jale	HAH leh
push	puje	POO heh
bend	dóblese	DOH vleh seh
open	abra	AH vrah
close	cierre	SYEH rreh
episiotomy	episiotomía	eh pee syoh toh MEE ah
stitches	puntos	POON tohs

Breathe deeply.
Respire profundamente.
rrehs PEE reh proh foon dah MEHN teh

Squeeze this.
Apriete esto.
ah PRYEH teh_EHS toh

Move your leg.
Mueva la pierna.
MWEH vah lah PYEHR nah

Raise your head.
Levante la cabeza.
leh VAHN teh lah kah VEH sah

Rest.
Descanse.
dehs KAHN seh

This is for the pain.
Esto es para el dolor.
EHS toh_ehs PAH rah_ehl thoh LOHR

You need anesthesia.
Necesita anestesia.
neh seh SEE tah_ah nehs TEH syah

You need a Cesarean section.
Necesita una operación cesárea.
neh seh SEE tah_OO nah_oh peh rah SYOHN seh
SAH reh ah

Birth

It is a ...   Es ...   ehs

  boy.   un niño.   oon NEE nyoh

  girl.   una niña.   OO nah NEE nyah

He (she) is healthy.
Es sano (a).
ehs SAH noh (SAH nah)

Complications

There is a problem.
Hay un problema.
ay oom proh VLEH mah

I'm sorry to tell you this.
Siento decirle esto.
SYEHN toh theh SEER leh_EHS toh

The baby has a birth defect.
El bebé tiene un defecto de nacimiento.
ehl veh VEH TYEH neh_oon theh FEHK toh
theh nah see MYEHN toh

The baby is jaundiced.
El bebé tiene ictericia.
ehl veh VEH TYEH neh_eek teh REE syah

The baby was stillborn.
El bebé nació muerto.
ehl veh VEH nah SYOH MWEHR toh

You've had a miscarriage.
Ha tenido un aborto espontáneo.
ah teh NEE thoh_oon ah VOHR toh_ehs pohn
TAH neh oh

Postpartum

Call the doctor if you or the baby has a fever.
Llame al médico si usted o el bebé tiene fiebre.
YAH meh_ahl MEH thee koh see_oos TEHTH
oh_ehl veh VEH TYEH neh FYEH vreh

You should wait six weeks to have intercourse.
No debe tener relaciones sexuales por seis semanas.
noh THEH veh teh NEHR rreh lah SYOH nehs
sehk SWAH lehs pohr seys seh MAH nahs

Call this number for breastfeeding problems and
questions.
Llame a este número si tiene algún problema o duda.
YAH meh_ah_EHS teh NOO meh roh see TYEH
neh_ahl GOOM proh VLEH mah_oh THOO thah

Menopause

When the reproductive years end, women face a
whole new set of health issues. Here are the
phrases you'll need to discuss them:

Are you having your periods ...
¿Ha notado que tiene la regla ...
ah noh TAH thoh keh TYEH neh lah RREH glah

> more often?
> más frecuentemente?
> mahs freh kwehn teh MEHN teh

less often?
menos frecuentemente?
MEH nohs freh kwehn teh MEHN teh

Are your periods …
¿Nota que su regla …
NOH tah keh soo RREH glah

heavier?
tiene más sangre?
TYEH neh mahs SAHN greh

lighter?
tiene menos sangre?
TYEH neh MEH nohs SAHN greh

You are going through menopause.
Está pasando por la menopausia.
ehs TAH pah SAHN doh pohr lah meh noh POW
syah

This is normal.
Esto es normal.
EHS toh_ehs nohr MAHL

Most symptoms will pass by themselves.
La mayoría de los síntomas desaparecen solos.
lah mah yoh REE ah theh lohs SEEN toh mahs
theh sah pah REH sehn SOH lohs

I can give you something to make you more
comfortable.
Puedo darle algo para que esté más a gusto.
PWEH thoh THAHR leh_AHL goh PAH rah
keh_ehs TEH mahs ah GOOS toh

12

Emergencies

People tend to get emotional in emergencies, and that can interfere with the exchange of vital information you need to provide timely care. When not everyone speaks the same language, it gets even harder to exchange information quickly and efficiently.

In a medical emergency involving Spanish speakers, it's likely the patient will be surrounded by an army of friends and family or well-meaning witnesses, all eager to voice their feelings and tell you what happened. As you listen, don't equate the volume and speed of their speech with impatience or anger. It's just heightened emotion. To gain control of the situation and get the information you need, stay very calm and say that your Spanish is not good enough for you to understand them when they speak that way:

> I'm sorry but my Spanish isn't good enough for me to understand you when you talk that way.
> Perdone, lo siento, pero mi español ne me vale cuando usted habla así.
> pehr THOH neh, loh SYEHN toh, PEH roh mee_ehs pah NYOHL noh meh VAH leh KWAHN doh_oos TEHTH AH vlah_ah SEE

If you display heroic calm and admit the limitations of your Spanish, family, friends, and well-meaning witnesses will understand that to help you help their loved one, they need to settle down. With order restored, you can take care of the patient.

Words for When Time Counts

With Spanish speakers, it's usually best to make requests gently, and with deference. In an emergency, however, you may need to cast your requests as commands. Here are some of the most useful:

Breathe.
Respire.
rrehs PEE reh

Breathe more slowly.
Respire más despacio.
rrehs PEE reh mahs thehs PAH syoh

Close your eyes.
Cierre los ojos.
SYEH rreh lohs OH hohs

Follow instructions.
Siga las instrucciones.
SEE gah lahs eens trook SYOH nehs

Follow me.
Sígame.
SEE gah meh

Follow my finger.
Siga mi dedo.
SEE gah mee theh thoh

Help me.
Ayúdeme.
ah YOO theh meh

Lie still.
Estése quieto.
ehs TEH seh KYEH toh

Listen.
Escuche.
ehs KOO cheh

Look at me.
Míreme.
MEE reh meh

Look here.
Mire aquí.
MEE reh ah KEE

Lower your head.
Baje la cabeza.
BAH heh lah kah VEH sah

Open your eyes.
Abra los ojos.
AH vrah lohs OH hohs

Open your mouth.
Abra la boca.
AH vrah lah VOH kah

Raise your arm.
Levante el brazo.
leh VAHN teh_ehl BRAH soh

Raise your leg.
Levante la pierna.
leh VAHN teh lah PYEHR nah

Say "ah."
Diga "aaaah."
DEE gah aaaaaaah

Sit up.
Incorpórese.
een kohr POH reh seh

Squeeze my hand.
Apriete mi mano.
ah PREYH teh mee MAH noh

Stand on your heels.
Párese en los talones.
PAH reh seh_ehn lohs tah LOH nehs

Stand on your toes.
Párese en los dedos de los pies.
PAH reh seh_ehn lohs THEH thohs theh lohs pyehs

Swallow this.
Trague esto.
TRAH geh_EHS toh

Tell me.
Dígame.
DEE gah meh

Touch your nose.
Tóquese la nariz.
TOH keh seh lah nah REES

Turn over.
Dése vuelta. / Vuélvase.
DEH seh VWEHL tah / VWEHL vah seh

Turn your head.
Vuelva la cabeza.
VWEHL vah kah VEH

Walk like this.
Camine así.
kah MEE neh_ah SEE

For First Responders

In an emergency, hospital staff need to ask questions and give instructions quickly and efficiently. But so do the people at the scene of an emergency. Police, fire, ambulance, and EMT health-care professionals have just as much need to communicate swiftly, and perhaps more.

In an emergency, you need to find out what happened and who needs your immediate attention, and keep the situation calm. When it involves Spanish speakers, here are a few words you might hear:

Danger!	¡Peligro!	peh LEE groh
Fire!	¡Fuego!	FWEH goh
Help!	¡Socorro!	soh KOH rroh

To identify yourself, say the following:

Hi, I'm with the ...
Hola, trabajo con ...
OH lah, trah VAH hoh kohn

fire department.
los bomberos.
lohs bohm BEH rohs

police department.
la policía.
lah poh lee SEE ah

ambulance service.
la ambulancia.
lah_ahm boo LAHN syah

Through Their Eyes

Even in an emergency, begin with a polite standard greeting, like *Buenos días* (Hello), to put the patient, family, and friends at ease.

And to offer reassurance:

I'm here to help you.
Estoy aquí para ayudarle.
ehs TOY ah KEE PAH rah_ah yoo THAHR leh

What is your name?
¿Cómo se llama?
KOH moh seh YAH mah

You will be okay.
Todo estará bien.
TOH thoh_ehs tah RAH veyhn

The ambulance is on its way.
La ambulancia está en camino.
lah_ahm boo LAHN syah_ehs TAH_ehn kah
MEE noh

We're taking you to the hospital.
Vamos a llevarle al hospital.
VAH mohs ah yeh VAHR leh_ahl ohs pee TAHL

I will notify your family.
Notificaré a su familia.
noh tee fee kah REH_ah soo fah MEE lyah

And for family and friends with the patient:

Please stay calm.
Cálmense.
KAHL mehn seh

Please wait here.
Esperen aquí.
ehs PEH rehn ah KEE

The doctor is coming.
Ya viene el médico.
yah VYEH neh_ehl MEH thee koh

The nurse is coming.
Ya viene la enfermera.
yah VYEH neh lah_ehn fehr MEH rah

We are working on her (him) now.
Estamos atendiendola (lo) ahora mismo.
ehs TAH mohs ah tehn DYEHN doh lah (loh)_ah
OH rah MEES moh

What Happened?

Whether in the field or in the emergency room,
you'll want to find out exactly what happened so you

know what you're dealing with. If the patient can't answer these questions, you can address them to observers:

Was there …
¿Hubo …
OO voh

an accident?	un accidente?	oon ahk see THEHN teh
an assault?	un asalto?	oon ah SAHL toh
chest pain (pressure)?	dolor (presión) en el pecho?	thoh LOHR (preh SYOHN) ehn ehl PEH choh
a dog bite?	una mordedura de perro?	OO na mohr theh THOO rah theh PEH rroh
a fall?	una caída?	OO nah kah EE thah
an insect bite?	una picadura de insecto?	OO nah pee kah THOO rah theh_een SEHK toh
an overdose?	una sobredosis?	OO nah soh vreh THOH sees
a seizure?	un ataque convulsivo?	oon ah TAH keh kohm bool SEE voh
dizziness?	mareos?	mah REH ohs

Were you (was the patient) exposed to extreme cold?
¿Se expuso (el paciente) a un frío intenso?
seh_ehs POO soh_(ehl pah SYEHN teh)_ah_oon FREE oh_een tehn SEE voh

Did you (did the patient) faint or get nauseated from the heat?

¿Se desmayó o tuvo náuseas (el paciente) debido al calor?

seh thehs mah YOH_oh TOO voh NOW seh ahs (ehl pah SYEHN teh) theh VEE thoh_ahl kah LOHR

¡Ojo!

Remember, you need learn only one verb form for he, she, it, and you.

When you talk *to* the patient, the verb automatically means "you," when you talk *about* the patient, it means "he" or "she," and when you talk about something, it means "it."

Were you (was the patient) hurt by some object?

¿Le hizo daño (al paciente) algo?

leh_EE soh thah nyoh (ehl pah SYEHN teh)_AHL goh

Were you (was the patient) shot?

¿Se le pegó un tiro (al paciente)?

seh leh peh GOH_oon TEE roh_(ahl pah SYEHN teh)

Were you (was the patient) raped?

¿Fue violada (la paciente)?

fweh vyoh LAH thah (lah pah SYEHN teh)

How much have you (has the patient) had to drink today?
¿Cuánto ha tomado (el paciente) hoy?
KWAHN toh_ah toh MAH thoh_(ehl pah SYEHN teh)_oy

Over the Phone

In an emergency, you'll need to establish certain things right away. Here are some vital questions and instructions to use if you're talking to someone on the phone:

What is your injury?
¿Qué herida tiene?
keh_eh REE thah TYEH neh

Can you move?
¿Puede moverse?
PWEH theh moh VEHR seh

Are you bleeding?
¿Está sangrando?
ehs TAH sahn GRAHN doh

Are you burned?
¿Se ha quemado?
seh_ah keh MAH thoh

Do you think anything is broken?
¿Cree que se ha roto algo?
KREH eh keh seh_ah RROH toh_AHL goh

Are you pregnant?
¿Está embarazada?
ehs TAH_ehm bah rah SAH thah

Are you in labor?
¿Ya comenzó el parto?
yah koh mehn SOH_ehl PAHR toh

Is anyone with you?
¿Hay otra persona con usted?
ay OH trah pehr SOH nah kohn oos TEHTH

Call this number ___.
Llame a este número ___.
YAH meh_ah_EHS teh NOO meh roh

Come to the hospital immediately.
¡Venga inmediatamente al hospital!
BEHN gah_een meh thyah tah MEHN teh_ahl ohs
pee TAHL

In the ER

When assessing a patient in the emergency room,
many of the previous questions are still useful. But
you'll also want to ask others.

Pain

Many patients arrive in the ER in considerable pain.
For in-depth help in assessing it, see Chapter 5.

Abuse and Assault

When it's obvious a patient is the victim of abuse or
assault, or you only suspect it, see Chapter 5 for the
questions to ask.

Illness

When the emergency stems from an illness, not trauma, the questions you'll ask are a bit different.

(For the Spanish names of many illnesses, see Chapter 7. For phrases to use in taking a detailed history, see Chapter 4, and for the words to use when performing a physical exam, see Chapter 5.)

What illness do you have?
¿Qué enfermedad tiene?
keh_ehn fehr meh THAHTH TYEH neh

How old are you?
¿Cuántos años tiene?
KWAHN tohs AH nyohs TYEH neh

Has this happened before?
¿Le ha pasado esto antes?
leh_ah pah SAH thoh_EHS toh_AHN tehs

Does this happen a lot?
¿Le pasa esto mucho?
leh PAH sah_EHS toh MOO choh

Are you under a doctor's care?
¿Está bajo el cuidado de un doctor?
ehs TAH VAH hoh_ehl kwee THAH thoh theh_oon thohk TOHR

What is his (her) name?
¿Cómo se llama él (ella)?
KOH moh seh YAH mah_ehl (EH yah)

Where can I reach her (him)?
¿Cómo puedo comunicarme con él (ella)?
KOH moh PWEH thoh koh moo nee KAHR meh
kohn ehl (EH yah)

What medications are you currently taking?
¿Qué medicinas toma actualmente?
keh meh thee SEE nahs TOH mah ahk twahl
MEHN teh

Do you have them with you?
¿Las trae consigo?
lahs TRAH eh kohn SEE goh

May I see them?
¿Puedo verlas?
PWEH thoh VEHR lahs

Are you allergic to any medicines?
¿Tiene alergia a cualquier medicina?
TYEH neh_ah LEHR hyah_ah kwahl KYEHR
meh thee SEE nah

Burns

When a patient has burns, you may want to know
their source:

How were you (was the patient) burned?
¿Cómo se quemó (el paciente)?
KOH moh seh keh MOH (ehl pah SYEHN teh)

The answer will be one of the following:

chemicals	los productos químicos	lohs proh THOOK tohs KEE mee kohs
electricity	la electricidad	lah_eh lehk tree see THAHTH
fireworks	los fuegos artificiales	lohs FWEH gohs ahr tee fee SYAH lehs
flames	las llamas	lahs YAH mahs
heat	el calor	ehl kah LOHR
scalding	la escaldadura	lah ehs kahl thah THOO rah
hot water	el agua caliente	ehl AH gwah kah LYEHN the
grease	la grasa	lah GRAH sah
oil	el aceite	ehl ah SEY the
radiation	la radiación	lah rrah thyah SYOHN

Head Injuries

If the patient is unconscious, he or she will likely be sent directly to Intensive Care. If the patient has a head injury but is conscious, use these questions to perform your assessment:

I'm going to ask you some simple questions.
Voy a hacerle unas preguntas sencillas.
boy ah_ah SEHR leh_OO nahs preh GOON tahs sehn SEE yahs

What is your name?
¿Cómo se llama?
KOH moh seh YAH mah

Where are you?
¿Dónde está?
DOHN deh_ehs TAH

What is the date?
¿Cuál es la fecha?
kwahl ehs lah FEH chah

Who is the president now?
¿Quién es el presidente?
kyehn ehs ehl preh see THEHN teh

What is happening in this room right now?
¿Qué pasa ahora mismo en esta sala?
keh PAH sah_ah OH rah MEES moh_ehn EHS tah
SAH lah

How many of my fingers do you see?
¿Cuántos dedos me ve?
KWAHN tohs THEH thohs meh veh

Squeeze my fingers with both hands.
Apriete mis dedos con las dos manos.
ah PRYEH teh mees THEH thohs kohn lahs thohs
MAH nohs

Do you have a headache?
¿Le duele la cabeza?
leh THWEH leh lah kah VEH sah

Were you knocked out?
¿Perdió el conocimiento?
pehr THYOH_ehl koh noh see MYEHN toh

How long were you unconscious?
¿Cuánto tiempo quedó sin conocimiento?
KWAHN toh TYEHM poh keh thoh SEEN koh
noh see MYEHN toh

Did you see stars?
¿Vio centellos?
Byoh sehn TEH yohs

Do you feel nauseated?
¿Tiene náuseas?
TYEH neh NOW seh ahs

I'm sorry; due to your head injury, we cannot give
you pain medication.
Lo siento; debido a la herida de su cabeza, no
podemos darle medicina para el dolor.
loh SYEHN toh; theh VEE thoh_ah lah_eh REE
thah theh soo kah VEH sah, noh poh THEH mohs
THAHR leh meh thee SEE nah PAH rah_ehl thoh
LOHR

Poisoning and Drug Overdose

When an emergency results from something
ingested, ask the following:
What did you (he, she) ...
¿Qué ...
keh ...

drink?	tomó?/bebió?	toh MOH/ veh VYOH
eat?	comió?	koh MYOH
swallow?	tragó?	trah GOH

How long ago did you (he, she) swallow it?
¿Cuánto hace que lo tragó?
KWAHN toh_AH seh keh loh trah GOH

How much did you (he, she) swallow?
¿Cuánto tragó?
KWAHN toh trah GOH

The answer might be alcohol, a household product,
an over-the-counter or prescription medication
taken improperly, or even food:

alcohol	el alcohol	el ahl koh OHL
ammonia	el amoníaco	ehl ah moh NEE ah koh
amphetamines	las anfetaminas	lahs ahn feh tah MEE nahs
antihistamines	antihistaminas	ahn tee_ees tah MEE nahs
antiseptics	antisépticos	ahn tee SEHP tee kohs
aspirin	aspirina	ahs pee REE nah
barbiturates	barbitúricos	bahr bee TOO ree kohs
bleach	la lejía/ el blanqueador/ el cloro	la leh HEE ah/ ehl blahn keh ah THOHR/ ehl KLOH roh
capsules	las cápsulas	lahs KAHP soo lahs
contraceptives	anticonceptivos	ahn tee kohn sehp TEE vohs
cough syrup	jarabe para la tos	hah RAH vhe PAH rah lah tohs
cyanide	el cianuro	ehl syah NOO roh

continues

continued

detergent	el detergente	ehl theh tehr HEHN teh
food	la comida	lah koh MEE thah
household cleaners	productos de limpieza	proh THOOK tohs theh leem PYEH sah
insecticide	el insecticida	ehl een sehk tee SEE thah
liquor	el licor	ehl lee KOHR
lye	la lejía	lah leh HEE ah
medicine	la medicina	lah meh thee SEE nah
mushrooms	los hongos	lohs OHN gohs
paint	la pintura	lah peen TOO rah
pills	las píldoras	lahs PEEL thoh rahs
poison	el veneno	ehl veh NEH noh
sleeping pills	los somníferos	lohs sohm NEE feh rohs
tablets	las tabletas/ las pastillas/ los comprimidos	lahs tah VLEH tahs/ lahs pahs TEE yahs/ lohs kohm pree MEE thohs
tranquilizers	los tranquil- izantes	lohs trahn kee lee SAHN tehs

¡Ojo!

Strangely, the everyday word for laundry bleach is *lejía*, which actually means lye. You can clarify using the other equally imprecise words above for whitener or chlorine.

It might also be a street drug:

amphetamines	las anfetaminas	lahs ahn feh tah MEE nahs
barbiturates	los barbitúricos	lohs vahr vee TOO ree kohs
cocaine	la cocaína/la coca	lah koh kah EE nah/lah KOH kah
crack	el crac	ehl krahk
glue	la goma, la cola	lah GOH mah, lah KOH lah
hashish	el hachich	ehl ah cheech
heroin	la heroína	lah eh roh EE nah
marijuana	la marihuana/ la mota/la hierba	lah mah ree WAH nah/lah MOH tah/ lah YEHR vah
morphine	la morfina	lah mohr FEE nah

If you're giving instructions over the phone, depending on the circumstances, you might say:

Drink ...   Tome ...   TOH meh ...

milk	leche	LEH cheh
egg whites	claras de huevos	KLAH rahs theh WEH vohs
vinegar	vinagre	vee NAH greh
strong tea	té fuerte	teh FWEHR teh
black coffee	café negro	kah FEH NEH groh
mineral oil	aceite mineral	ah SEY teh mee neh RAHL
antacid	antiácido	ahn TYAH see thoh

Induce vomiting with ...
Hágase vomitar con ...
AH gah seh voh mee TAHR kohn ...

your finger	su dedo	soo THEH thoh
mustard and water	agua con mostaza	AH gwah kohn mohs TAH sah
salt and water	agua con sal	AH gwah kohn sahl

Call 9-1-1.
Llame al nueve uno uno.
YAH meh_ahl NWEH VEH OO noh OO noh

Come to the hospital immediately.
Venga al hospital inmediatamente.
VEHN gah_ahl ohs pee TAHL een meh thyah tah MEHN teh

Diagnosis and Treatment

After you've examined the patient, the family will want to know their loved one's immediate status:

He (she) is going to be fine.
Va a salir bien.
BAH_ah sah LEER vyehn

He (she) is resting comfortably.
Está descansando tranquilamente.
ehs TAH thehs kahn SAHN doh trahn kee lah
MEHN teh

We've given him (her) something for the pain.
Le hemos dado algo para el dolor.
leh_EH mohs THAH thoh_AHL goh PAH
rah_ehl thoh LOHR

> He (she) is ...
> Está ...
> ehs TAH ...

conscious	consciente	kohn SYEHN teh
awake	despierto(a)	thehs PYEHR toh (tah)
alert	alerta	ah LEHR tah
unconscious	inconsciente	een kohn SYEHN teh
in a coma	en estado de coma	ehn ehs TAH thoh theh KOH mah

We are trying to resuscitate him (her).
Estamos tratando de resucitarlo (la).
ehs TAH mohs trah TAHN doh theh rreh soo see
TAHR loh (lah)

It's too soon to know anything.
Es demasiado pronto para saber.
ehs theh mah SYAH thoh PROHN toh PAH rah
sah VEHR

And everyone will want to know what you've found.
These are some diagnoses commonly made in the ER:

He (she) is ... / You are ...

Está ...

ehs TAH ...

> bleeding.
>
> sangrando.
>
> sahn GRAHN doh
>
> dehydrated.
>
> deshidratado(a).
>
> theh see thrah TAH thoh (thah)

You (he, she) has ...

Tiene ...

TYEH neh ...

a broken bone	un hueso fracturado	oon WEH soh frahk too RAH thoh
bruises	unos cardenales	OO nos kahr theh NAH lehs
burns	unas quemaduras	OO nahs keh mah THOO rahs
a concussion	un golpe fuerte a la cabeza	oon GOHL peh FWEHR teh_ah lah kah VEH sah
some cuts	unas cortadas	OO nahs kohr TAH thahs
a dislocation	un hueso salido	oon WEH soh sah LEE thoh
a drug overdose	una sobredosis/ una dosis excesiva	OO nah soh vreh THOH sees/ OO nah THOH sees ehk seh SEE vah

food poisoning	una intoxicación (alimenticia)	OO nah_een tohk see kah SYOHN (ah lee mehn TEE syah)
a fracture	una fractura	OO nah frahk TOO rah
frostbite	una quemadura por frío	OO nah keh mah THOO rah pohr FREE oh
heat stroke	una insolación	OO nah_een soh lah SYOHN
hypothermia	hipotermia	ee poh TEHR myah
indigestion (popular)	ardor en el estómago	ahr THOHR ehn ehl ehs TOH mah goh
lacerations	cortadas	kohr TAH thahs
poisoning	un envenenamiento	oon ehm beh neh nah MYEHN toh
punctures	perforaciones	pehr foh rah SYOH nehs
a sprain	una torcedura	OO nah tohr seh THOO rah

You (he, she) has had …
Ha tenido …
ah teh NEE thoh

    a stroke.
    una embolia.
    OO nah_ehm BOH lyah

    a heart attack.
    un ataque al corazón.
    oon ah TAH keh_ahl koh rah SOHN

And some common treatments and recommendations:

> You (he, she) need(s) …
> Necesita …
> neh seh SEE tah …

a bandage	una venda	OO nah VEHN dah
a blood transfusion	una transfusión de sangre	OO nah trans foo SYOHN deh SAHN greh
blood work	un análisis de sangre	oon ah NAH lee sees theh SAHN greh
a cast	un yeso	oon YEH soh
intensive care	cuidado intensivo	kwee THAH thoh_ een tehn SEE voh
intravenous fluids	líquidos intravenosos	LEE kee thohs een trah veh NOH sohs
medication	medicamentos	meh thee kah MEHN tohs
more tests	más pruebas	mahs PRWEH vahs
oxygen	el oxígeno	ehl ohk SEE heh noh
a shot	una inyección	OO nah_een yehk SYOHN
a sling	un cabestrillo	oon kah vehs TREE yoh
a splint	una férula	OO nah FEH roo lah
stitches	los puntos	loh POON tohs
surgery	cirugía	see roo HEE ah
to be admitted	internarse	een tehr NAHR seh
to see a specialist	ver a un especialista	vehr ah_oon ehs peh syah LEES tah

For the names of more illnesses and conditions, see Chapter 7. For more phrases that describe treatments, see Chapter 8.

Chapter 13

Mental Health

Communicating with English-speaking patients who have mental conditions can be difficult enough; when there's also a language barrier, it can be even more challenging. One approach that works well, especially with Hispanic patients, is to start by asking about events and their sequence only, as the patient experiences them. Don't ask about possible reasons for them just yet. And use common, everyday language—but not street slang—as much as possible, not technical terms.

For instance, instead of asking about "hallucinations," you might ask the following:

> What was it you saw, that you later realized wasn't there?
> ¿Qué fue lo que vio, que luego se dio cuenta que no estaba allí?
> keh fweh loh keh vyoh, keh LWEH goh seh thyoh KWEHN tah keh noh_ehs TAH vah_ah YEE

You may need to explore reasons later, but this careful, nonjudgmental approach will help you gain candid information and establish initial rapport with your Spanish-speaking patients, without jeopardizing their dignity.

Mental Health

It can take careful probing to properly assess the many different types and levels of disorders that affect mental health. The questions that follow cover some common mental health conditions and will help you make a diagnosis and determine a treatment plan.

Questions for All

These are some questions that apply in many if not most mental health scenarios:

How long have you been experiencing this?
¿Cuánto tiempo hace que le pasa esto?
KWAHN toh TYEHM poh AH seh keh leh PAH sah_EHS toh

¡Ojo!

To express duration in questions and answers "for [+ period of time]" use *hace [period of time] que [present tense verb]*, and to express time since "[time] ago" use *hace [tiempo] que [past tense verb]*.

(To understand your patient's reply, and get further information, see the words for numbers and periods of time in Chapter 2.)

As long as you can remember?
¿Siempre se ha sentido así?
SYEHM preh seh_ah sehn TEE thoh_ah SEE

Have you had these feelings for at least six months?
¿Hace por lo menos seis meses que se siente así?
AH seh pohr loh MEH nohs seys MEH sehs keh seh SYEHN teh_ah SEE

Have you experienced …
¿Ha experimentado …
ah_ehs peh ree mehn TAH thoh

> reduced appetite and weight loss?
> una reducción de apetito y peso?
> OO nah reh thook SYOHN theh_ah peh TEE toh_ee PEH soh

> increased appetite and weight gain?
> un aumento de apetito y de peso?
> oon ow MEHN toh theh_ah peh TEE toh_ee theh PEH soh

> trouble falling (staying) asleep?
> problema para dormirse (dormir sin interrupción)?
> proh VLEH mah PAH rah thohr MEER seh (thohr MEER seen een teh rroop SYOHN)

Has there been a change in your interest in …
¿Ha notado un cambio en su interés para …
ah noh TAH thoh_oon KAHM byoh_ehn soo_een
teh REHS PAH rah

> school?
> los estudios?
> lohs ehs TOO thyohs

> work?
> el trabajo?
> ehl trah VAH hoh

> family?
> la familia?
> lah fah MEE lyah

> dealing with other people?
> tratar con los demás?
> trah TAHR kohn lohs theh MAHS

> sexual relations?
> las relaciones sexuales?
> lahs rreh lah SYOH nehs sehk SWAH lehs

> music?
> la música?
> lah MOO see kah

> reading?
> leer?
> leh EHR

> shopping?
> ir de compras?
> eer theh KOHM prahs

> socializing?
> actividades sociales?
> ahk tee vee THAH thehs soh SYAH lehs

watching TV?
mirar la televisión?
mee RAHR lah teh leh vee SYOHN

other everyday activities?
otras actividades rutinarias?
OH trahs ahk tee vee THAH thehs roo tee
NAH ryahs

Do you have trouble concentrating?
¿Tiene problemas para concentrarse?
TYEH neh proh VLEH mahs PAH rah kohn sehn
TRAHR seh

Have you been treated by a doctor for this problem
before?
¿Ha recibido tratamiento médico por este problema
antes?
ah rreh see VEE thoh trah tah MYEHN toh MEH
thee koh pohr EHS teh proh VLEH mah_AHN tehs

Did something bad happen before you started feeling this way,
¿Ocurrió algo malo justo antes de que usted
comenzara a sentirse así,
oh koo RRYOH_AHL goh MAH loh HOOS
toh_AHN tes theh keh_oos TEHTH koh mehn
SAH rah_ah sehn TEER seh_ah SEE,

   ... such as a death, a divorce, or a job loss?
   ... algo como una muerte, un divorcio, o el
   despido del trabajo?
   ... AHL goh KOH moh_OO nah MWEHR
   teh oon dee VOHR syoh, oh_ehl thehs PEE
   thoh thehl trah VAH hoh

Have you been hospitalized for this problem before?
¿Se ha hospitalizado antes por este problema?
seh_ah_ohs pee tah lee SAH thoh_AHN tehs pohr
EHS teh proh VLEH mah

Anxiety

Do you regularly have periods when you feel
extremely nervous (anxious)?
¿Le vienen a menudo períodos cuando se siente
excesivamente nervioso(a) o ansioso(a)?
leh VYEH nehn ah meh NOO thoh peh REE oh
thohs KWAHN doh seh SYEHN teh_ehk seh see
vah MEHN teh nehr VYOH soh (sah)_ohahn
SYOH soh (sah)

Are you troubled by excessive worry about ...
¿Se preocupa excesivamente por ...
seh preh oh KOO pah_ehk seh see vah MEHN teh
pohr

> your health?
> la salud?
> lah sah LOOTH
>
> school?
> los estudios?
> lohs ehs TOO thyohs
>
> work?
> el trabajo?
> ehl trah VAH hoh

Do you feel unable to control the worry?
¿Se siente incapaz de controlar su preocupación?
seh SYEHN teh_een kah PAHS theh kohn troh
LAHR soo preh oh koo pah SYOHN

Do you get tired easily?
¿Se cansa fácilmente?
seh KAHN sah FAH seel MEHN teh

Do you feel restless?
¿Se inquieta por todo?
seh_een KYEH tah pohr TOH thoh

Do you feel irritable?
¿Se irrita por todo?
seh_ee RREE tah pohr TOH thoh

During the periods you feel extremely nervous, do
you ...
Cuando se pone muy nervioso(a), ¿tiene usted ...
KWAHN doh seh POH neh muy nehr VYOH soh
(sah), TYEH neh_oos TEHTH

> have muscle tension?
> tensión en los músculos?
> tehn SYOHN ehn lohs MOOS koo lohs
>
> have a dry mouth?
> la boca seca?
> lah VOH kah SEH kah
>
> get dizzy or light-headed?
> mareos?
> mah REH ohs
>
> feel your heart beat fast?
> palpitaciones del corazón?
> pahl pee tah SYOH nehs thehl koh rah SOHN
>
> feel like you can't catch your breath?
> la sensación de que le falta aire?
> lah sehn sah SYOHN theh keh leh FAHL
> tah_AY reh

feel you can't swallow?
dificultad para tragar?
thee fee kool TAHTH PAH rah trah GAHR

How long do these periods last?
¿Cuánto duran estos períodos?
KWAHN toh THOO rahn EHS tohs peh REE oh
thohs

Do you regularly feel …
¿Con frecuencia se siente …
kohn keh freh KWEHN syah seh SYEHN teh

> sad?
> triste?
> TREES teh
>
> depressed?
> deprimido(a)?
> theh pree MEE thoh (thah)
>
> disinterested in life?
> sin interés en la vida?
> seen een teh REHS ehn lah VEE thah
>
> guilty?
> culpable?
> kool PAH vleh
>
> worthless?
> sin valor?
> seen vah LOHR

Do you repeat certain activities to reduce your
distress?
¿Repite ciertas actividades para aliviar su angustia?
rreh PEE teh SYEHR tahs ahk tee vee THAH
thehs PAH rah_ah lee VYAHR soo_ahn GOOS tyah

Do you do things—such as wash your hands or lock doors—a particular number of times to keep something bad from happening?

¿Hay cosas que usted haga cierto número de veces para evitar que pase algo malo?

ay KOH sahs keh_oos TEHTH AH gah SYEHR toh NOO meh roh theh VEH sehs PAH rah_eh vee TAHR keh PAH seh_AHL goh MAH loh

Depression

Do you regularly feel …

¿Es común que usted se siente …

ehs koh MOON keh_oos TEHTH seh SYEHN teh

> anxious?
>
> ansioso(a)?
>
> ahn SYOH soh (sah)

> apathetic? (as if nothing matters)
>
> apático(a)? (que no le importa nada)
>
> ah PAH tee koh (kah) (keh noh leh_eem POHR tah NAH thah)

> "empty"?
>
> vacío(a)?
>
> vah SEE oh (ah)

> irritable?
>
> irritable?
>
> ee rree TAH vleh

> tearful?
>
> lagrimoso?
>
> lah gree MOH soh

When something good happens, do you feel happy?
Cuando pasa algo bueno, ¿se siente contento(a)?
KWAHN doh PAH sah_AHL goh VWEH noh,
seh SYEHN teh kohn TEHN toh (tah)

Emotionally, do you experience extreme highs and
extreme lows?
En cuanto a sus emociones, ¿experimenta usted
muchos altibajos?
ehn KWAHN toh_ah soos eh moh SYOH nehs,
ehs peh ree MEHN tah_oos TEHTH MOO chohs
ahl tee VAH hohs

Do you have difficulty making decisions?
¿Tiene dificultad para tomar decisiones?
TYEH neh thee fee kool TAHTH PAH rah toh
MAHR theh see SYOH nehs

Do you regularly feel …
Por lo común, ¿se siente …
pohr loh koh MOON, seh SYEHN teh

> guilty?
> culpable?
> kool PAH vleh

> badly about yourself?
> avergonzado(a) de sí mismo(a)?
> ah vehr gohn SAH thoh (thah) theh see MEES
> moh (mah)

> hopeless about your future?
> sin esperanza para el futuro?
> seen ehs peh RAHN sah PAH rah_ehl foo
> TOO roh

> worthless?
> que usted no vale nada?
> keh oos TEHTH noh VAH leh NAH thah

Harmful Tendencies

In some patients, mental problems can precipitate harmful actions. These are some questions to ask if you feel your patient is a risk to him- or herself, or to others.

Self

Do you regularly ...
Por lo común, ¿se encuentra ...
pohr loh koh MOON, seh_ehn KWEHN trah

> think of ways to harm yourself?
> pensando en maneras de hacerse daño?
> pehn SAHN doh_ehn mah NEH rahs theh_ah SEHR seh THAH nyoh

> think of ways to kill yourself (commit suicide)?
> pensando en maneras de matarse (suicidarse)?
> pehn SAHN doh_ehn mah NEH rahs theh mah TAHR seh (swee see THAHR seh)

> think about dying?
> pensando en la muerte?
> pehn SAHN doh_ehn lah MWEHR teh

> wish you were dead?
> deseando morirse?
> theh seh AHN doh moh REER seh

> feel others would be better off if you were dead?
> creyendo que los demás estarían mejor si usted muriera?
> kreh YEHN doh keh lohs theh MAHS ehs tah REE ahn meh HOHR see oos TEHTH moo RYEH rah

Have you attempted to harm or kill yourself before?
¿Ha intentado hacerse daño o matarse alguna vez?
ah_een tehn TAH thoh_ah SEHR seh THAH
nyoh_oh mah TAHR seh_ahl GOO nah vehs

Others

Do you have difficulty ...
¿Le es difícil ...
leh_ehs thee FEE seel

> controlling impulses?
> controlar sus impulsos?
> kohn troh LAHR soos eem POOL sohs

> controlling unpleasant feelings, such as anger?
> controlar emociones desagradables como la rabia?
> kohn troh LAHR eh moh SYOH nehs theh sah
> grah THAH vlehs KOH moh lah RRAH vyah

Do you have thoughts about harming someone else?
Who?
¿Ha pensado en hacerle daño a otra persona? ¿A
quién?
ah pehn SAH thoh_ehn ah SEHR leh THAH
nyoh_ah_OH trah pehr SOH nah ah kyehn

Have you harmed someone previously?
¿Le ha hecho daño a otra persona antes?
leh_ah_EH choh THAH nyoh_ah_OH trah pehr
SOH nah_AHN tehs

Do you have access to weapons?
¿Tiene acceso a las armas?
TYEH neh_ahk SEH soh_ah lahs AHR mahs

Have you ever been charged with assault or homicide?
¿Le han acusado de asalto u homicidio?
leh_ahn ah koo SAH thoh theh_ah SAHL
toh_oo_oh mee SEE thyoh

Mania

Emotionally, do you experience extreme highs and
extreme lows?
En cuanto a sus emociones, ¿experimenta usted
muchos altibajos?
ehn KWAHN toh_ah soos eh moh SYOH nehs, ehs
peh ree MEHN tah_oos TEHTH MOO chohs ahl
tee VAH hohs

Do you feel ...
¿Se siente usted ...
seh SYEHN teh_oos TEHTH

    happier than usual?
    más feliz que lo normal?
    mahs feh LEES keh loh nohr MAHL

    irritable?
    irritable?
    ee rree TAH vleh

    overly excited?
    excesivamente agitado(a)?
    ehk seh see vah MEHN teh_ah hee TAH thoh
    (thah)

    on top of the world?
    encima del mundo?
    ehn SEE mah thehl MOON doh

easily distracted by sights and sounds?
distraído(a) fácilmente por lo que oye y ve?
thees trah ee thoh (thah) FAH seel MEHN teh
pohr loh keh_OH yeh_ee veh

that there is nothing you can't do?
que no hay nada que no pueda hacer?
keh noh_ay NAH thah keh noh PWEH thah_ah
SEHR

Do you have more energy than usual?
¿Tiene más energía de lo normal?
TYEH neh mahs eh nehr HEE ah theh loh nohr
MAHL

Do you need less sleep lately?
Últimamente, ¿necesita dormir menos que antes?
OOL tee mah MEHN teh, neh seh SEE tah thohr
MEER MEH nohs keh_AHN tehs

Have you been …
¿Ha notado que …
ah noh TAH thoh keh

more talkative than usual?
es más hablador(a) que de costumbre?
ehs mahs ah vlah THOHR (THOH rah) keh
theh kohs TOOM breh

taking on more activities than usual?
emprende más actividades que de costumbre?
ehm PREHN deh mahs ahk tee vee THAH
thehs keh theh kohs TOOM breh

unable to concentrate because of racing thoughts?
no puede concentrarse porque se le acumulan los
pensamientos?
noh PWEH theh kohn sehn TRAHR seh pohr
keh seh leh_ah coo MOO lahn lohs pehn sah
MYEHN tohs

Are you ...
¿Está ...
ehs TAH

working more?
trabajando más?
trah vah HAHN doh mahs

spending more money?
gastando dinero sin pensar?
gahs TAHN doh thee NEH roh seen pehn SAHR

acting impulsively and doing reckless things?
comportándose insensata e impulsivamente?
kohm pohr TAHN doh seh_een sehn SAH
tah_eh_eem pool see vah MEHN teh

Have you ever been diagnosed with bipolar disorder?
¿Le han hecho una diagnosis de desorden bipolar?
leh_ahn EH choh_OO nah thyahg NOH sees theh
theh SOHR thehm bee poh LAHR

Did you stop taking your medications?
¿Ha dejado de tomar sus medicamentos?
ah theh HAH thoh theh toh MAHR soos meh thee
kah MEHN tohs

Schizophrenia

There are three common symptoms in people with schizophrenia that require treatment: anxiety, depression, and psychosis. The questions to ask about the first two are in their own sections above. The questions about psychosis are here:

Are you hearing voices in your head?
¿Oye voces en su mente?
OH yeh VOH sehs ehn soo MEHN teh

What are they saying to you?
¿Qué le están diciendo?
keh leh_ehs TAHN dee SYEHN doh

Do you feel as if the world is against you, or people are out to hurt you?
¿Se le hace que el mundo está en contra suyo, o que los demás desean hacerle daño?
seh leh_AH seh keh_ehl MOON doh_ehs
TAH_ehn KOHN trah SOO yoh, oh keh lohs theh
MAHS theh SEH ahn ah SEHR leh THAH nyoh

Has this happened before?
¿Le ha pasado esto antes?
leh_ah pah SAH thoh_EHS toh_AHN tehs

Did you get medication?
¿Le han dado medicamentos?
leh_ahn DAH thoh meh thee kah MEHN tohs

Did you stop taking it?
¿Ha dejado de tomarlos?
ah theh HAH thoh the toh MAHR lohs

Index

A

F

J-K-L

M

Q-R